Metabolic Confusion Diet Cookbook for Endomorph Women

The 7 Essential Pillars to Transform Your Body from Endomorph to Ectomorph.

Includes 4 Adaptive Meal Plans for Any Scenario

Jane Manson

Jane Manson © Copyright 2024. All rights reserved.

The content contained within this book may not be reproduced, duplicated, or transmitted without direct written permission from the author or the publisher.
Under no circumstances will any blame or legal responsibility be held against the publisher, or author, for any damages, reparation, or monetary loss due to the information contained within this book, either directly or indirectly.

Legal Notice:
This book is copyright-protected. It is only for personal use. You cannot amend, distribute, sell, use, quote or paraphrase any part, or the content within this book, without the consent of the author or publisher.

Disclaimer Notice:
Please note the information contained within this document is for educational and entertainment purposes only. All effort has been executed to present accurate, up-to-date, reliable, and complete information. No warranties of any kind are declared or implied. Readers acknowledge that the author is not engaging in the rendering of legal, financial, medical or professional advice. The content within this book has been derived from various sources. Please consult a licensed professional before attempting any techniques outlined in this book.

By reading this document, the reader agrees that under no circumstances is the author responsible for any losses, direct or indirect, that are incurred as a result of the use of the information contained within this document, including, but not limited to, errors, omissions, or inaccuracies.

Table of Contents

WELCOME MESSAGE	**9**
The Journey Ahead: What to Expect from This Book	9
Understanding Body Types: Endomorph vs. Mesomorph vs. Ectomorph	9
CHAPTER 1: UNDERSTANDING YOUR BODY TYPE	**11**
What is an Endomorph?	11
Characteristics and Traits	11
Common Challenges Faced by Endomorphs	12
What is a Mesomorph?	13
Characteristics and Traits	14
Benefits of Transitioning to a Mesomorph Body Type	15
What is an Ectomorph?	16
Characteristics and Traits	17
Benefits of Transitioning to an Ectomorph Body Type	18
The Science Behind Metabolism	19
Metabolic Rates and Hormonal Influence	20
How Metabolic Confusion Works	21
CHAPTER 2: THE METABOLIC CONFUSION DIET	**23**
Introduction to Metabolic Confusion	23
Definition and Principles	23
Benefits of Metabolic Confusion for Endomorphs	24
Calorie Cycling Explained	25
High-Calorie vs. Low-Calorie Days	26
Sample Calorie Cycling Schedules	27
Macronutrient Management	29
Importance of Protein, Carbs, and Fats	30
Adjusting Macronutrient Ratios for Optimal Results	31
CHAPTER 3: 7 PILLARS TO TRANSITION FROM ENDOMORPH TO ECTOMORPH	**33**
Pillar 1: Personalized Nutrition	33
Crafting Your Meal Plans	33
Foods to Embrace and Avoid	34
Pillar 2: Mindfulness and Stress Management	36
Impact of Stress on Weight Loss	37
Techniques for Stress Reduction and Mindfulness	38

PILLAR 3: HORMONAL BALANCE	**39**
UNDERSTANDING HORMONES AND THEIR ROLE	39
NATURAL WAYS TO BALANCE HORMONES	40
PILLAR 4: FITNESS AND EXERCISE	**42**
BEST EXERCISES FOR ENDOMORPHS	42
COMBINING CARDIO AND STRENGTH TRAINING	44
PILLAR 5: SUSTAINABLE LIFESTYLE CHANGES	**46**
BUILDING HEALTHY HABITS	46
MAINTAINING CONSISTENCY	48
PILLAR 6: COMMUNITY AND SUPPORT	**49**
IMPORTANCE OF SOCIAL SUPPORT	50
HOW TO BUILD YOUR SUPPORT NETWORK	50
PILLAR 7: TRACKING AND ADJUSTING	**52**
MONITORING PROGRESS	53
MAKING ADJUSTMENTS TO STAY ON TRACK	54
CHAPTER 4: RECIPES FOR SUCCESS	**56**
LOW-CALORIE BREAKFAST RECIPES	**56**
AVOCADO AND EGG WHITE SCRAMBLE	56
BERRY PROTEIN SMOOTHIE	56
CHIA SEED PUDDING WITH ALMOND MILK	57
COTTAGE CHEESE AND BERRY BOWL	57
GREEK YOGURT WITH FLAXSEEDS AND BLUEBERRIES	58
KALE AND SPINACH SMOOTHIE	58
QUINOA BREAKFAST BOWL WITH VEGETABLES	59
QUINOA BREAKFAST BOWL WITH VEGETABLES	59
SCRAMBLED TOFU WITH SPINACH AND TOMATOES	60
ZUCCHINI AND CARROT PANCAKES	60
LOW-CALORIE LUNCH RECIPES	**61**
BAKED COD WITH ASPARAGUS	61
CHICKEN AND AVOCADO SALAD	61
CHICKPEA AND SPINACH STEW	62
GRILLED SALMON WITH QUINOA	62
LENTIL AND VEGETABLE SOUP	63
SHRIMP AND ZUCCHINI NOODLES	63
SPINACH AND FETA STUFFED PEPPERS	64
TOFU AND BROCCOLI STIR-FRY	64
TURKEY LETTUCE WRAPS	65
ZUCCHINI AND TOMATO SALAD	65
LOW-CALORIE DINNER RECIPES	**66**
BAKED LEMON HERB CHICKEN	66
CAULIFLOWER RICE STIR-FRY	66
GARLIC BUTTER SHRIMP WITH ASPARAGUS	67

GRILLED EGGPLANT WITH TAHINI SAUCE	67
HERB-CRUSTED TILAPIA	68
QUINOA STUFFED BELL PEPPERS	68
SPROUTS AND CHICKEN	69
SALMON AND AVOCADO SALAD	69
SPAGHETTI SQUASH WITH MARINARA SAUCE	70
LOW-CALORIE SNACKS AND DESSERTS RECIPES	**70**
APPLE SLICES WITH ALMOND BUTTER	70
BERRY CHIA PUDDING	71
CUCUMBER AND HUMMUS BITES	71
DARK CHOCOLATE DIPPED STRAWBERRIES	72
FROZEN YOGURT BLUEBERRY BITES	72
GREEK YOGURT WITH HONEY AND WALNUTS	73
KALE CHIPS	73
PROTEIN-PACKED ENERGY BALLS	74
SPICED ROASTED CHICKPEAS	74
ZUCCHINI MUFFINS	75
HIGH-CALORIE BREAKFAST RECIPES	**75**
AVOCADO TOAST WITH POACHED EGG	75
BANANA AND ALMOND BUTTER SMOOTHIE	76
BLUEBERRY OATMEAL WITH WALNUTS	76
GREEK YOGURT PARFAIT WITH GRANOLA AND HONEY	77
NUTTY BANANA PANCAKES	77
OVERNIGHT CHIA PUDDING WITH MIXED NUTS	78
QUINOA BREAKFAST BOWL WITH SPINACH AND AVOCADOS	78
SALMON AND CREAM CHEESE BAGEL	79
SCRAMBLED EGGS WITH SMOKED SALMON AND SPINACH	79
SWEET POTATO AND BLACK BEAN BREAKFAST BURRITO	80
HIGH-CALORIE LUNCH RECIPES	**80**
AVOCADO CHICKEN SALAD	80
BEEF AND SWEET POTATO STEW	81
CHICKEN PESTO PASTA	81
GRILLED CHEESE AND TOMATO SOUP	82
LENTIL AND QUINOA SALAD WITH FETA	82
SALMON AND AVOCADO RICE BOWL	83
SHRIMP AND AVOCADO TACOS	83
SPINACH AND RICOTTA STUFFED CHICKEN BREAST	84
TURKEY AND HUMMUS WRAP	84
VEGGIE AND HUMMUS WRAP	85
HIGH-CALORIE DINNER RECIPES	**85**
BAKED SALMON WITH QUINOA AND VEGGIES	85
BEEF STIR-FRY WITH BROCCOLI	86
CHICKEN ALFREDO WITH ZOODLES	86
GRILLED LAMB CHOPS WITH SWEET POTATO MASH	87
LENTIL AND VEGETABLE CASSEROLE	87

Pork Tenderloin with Apple and Sage	88
Quinoa-Stuffed Portobello Mushrooms	88
Shrimp and Avocado Salad	89
Spaghetti Squash with Meatballs	89
Stuffed Bell Peppers with Ground Turkey	90
High-Calorie Snacks and Desserts recipes	**90**
Almond Butter Energy Balls	90
Avocado Chocolate Mousse	91
Banana Walnut Bread	91
Dark Chocolate Almond Bark	92
Greek Yogurt with Honey and Granola	92
Nutty Apple Slices	93
Oatmeal Raisin Cookies	93
Peanut Butter and Banana Toast	94
Protein-Packed Smoothie Bowl	94
Sweet Potato Brownies	95
Plant-Based Recipes	**95**
Avocado and Black Bean Salad	95
Cauliflower Buffalo Wings	96
Chickpea and Spinach Curry	96
Grilled Portobello Mushrooms with Quinoa	97
Lentil and Vegetable Stew	97
Mixed Vegetable Stir-Fry with Tofu	98
Roasted Beet and Kale Salad	98
Spaghetti Squash with Tomato Basil Sauce	99
Sweet Potato and Black Bean Tacos	99
Zucchini Noodles with Pesto	100
Vegan and vegetarian Protein Recipes	**100**
Black Bean and Corn Salad	100
Chickpea and Spinach Stuffed Sweet Potatoes	101
Edamame and Quinoa Salad	101
Greek Yogurt and Berry Parfait	102
Lentil and Vegetable Stir-Fry	102
Protein-Packed Green Smoothie	103
Quinoa and Black Bean Stuffed Bell Peppers	103
Tofu and Vegetable Stir-Fry	104
Vegan Chickpea Omelette	104
White Bean and Kale Soup	105
CHAPTER 5: MEAL PLANS	**106**
Meal Plan 1: Basic Alternating Schedule	**106**
Meal Plan 2: 5:2 Schedule	**107**
Meal Plan 3: Fitness Enthusiast Schedule	**108**

MEAL PLAN 4: PROFESSIONAL AND BUSY LIFESTYLE SCHEDULE	109
CHAPTER 6: MINDFULNESS AND STRESS REDUCTION TECHNIQUES	**110**
INTRODUCTION TO MINDFULNESS	**110**
BENEFITS OF MINDFULNESS FOR WEIGHT LOSS	110
DAILY MINDFULNESS PRACTICES	111
STRESS MANAGEMENT STRATEGIES	**113**
BREATHING EXERCISES	113
GUIDED MEDITATIONS	115
JOURNALING AND REFLECTION	116
CONCLUSION	**119**

Thank you so much for purchasing my book! I'm thrilled to have you as part of my reading family.

If you could take a moment to scan the QR code below and leave your honest review on Amazon, I would be deeply grateful.

If you are reading the ebook version, please click on this link:

https://www.amazon.com/review/create-review?&ASIN=B0DB2JG238

Your feedback is incredibly important to me—it helps me grow as a writer and makes our community stronger. I genuinely love hearing from you and value your thoughts immensely!

Welcome Message

Welcome to the Metabolic Confusion Diet Cookbook for Endomorph Women. This comprehensive guide is meticulously crafted to address the unique needs and challenges faced by women with endomorphic body types. Grounded in scientific research and practical experience, my approach integrates the principles of metabolic confusion with tailored dietary and lifestyle strategies. Our goal is to empower you with the knowledge and tools necessary to achieve sustainable weight loss and improved health. Embark on this transformative journey with confidence, knowing that every step is supported by evidence-based insights and expert guidance. Let's begin this journey towards a healthier, more vibrant you.

The Journey Ahead: What to Expect from This Book

Embarking on a journey towards optimal health and weight management can be daunting, especially for women with an endomorphic body type. This book is designed to serve as your comprehensive guide, providing you with the necessary tools, knowledge, and strategies to successfully navigate the path of metabolic confusion dieting. Our approach is rooted in scientific evidence and practical application, ensuring that you receive accurate and actionable advice.

In this book, you will find a detailed exploration of the metabolic confusion diet, tailored specifically for endomorphic women. We will delve into the principles of calorie and macronutrient cycling, explaining how these strategies can be utilized to boost your metabolism, promote fat loss, and enhance overall well-being. You will learn how to implement these dietary changes in a way that fits seamlessly into your lifestyle, making it easier to adhere to the program and achieve lasting results.

Additionally, we will cover essential topics such as the importance of personalized nutrition, the role of exercise in supporting metabolic health, and the psychological aspects of weight management. Our practical tips, sample meal plans, and delicious recipes are designed to make your transition to this new way of eating as smooth and enjoyable as possible.

By the end of this book, you will be equipped with a deeper understanding of your body's unique needs and how to meet them through a balanced and scientifically-backed approach. We are committed to supporting you every step of the way, ensuring that you have the confidence and knowledge to transform your health and achieve your weight loss goals. Let's embark on this transformative journey together.

Understanding Body Types: Endomorph vs. Mesomorph vs. Ectomorph

The concept of somatotypes, or body types, was first introduced by Dr. William H. Sheldon in the 1940s. He categorized human bodies into three primary types: endomorph, mesomorph, and ectomorph. Each body type has distinct characteristics, metabolic tendencies, and nutritional needs, which can significantly impact one's approach to diet and exercise. Understanding these differences is crucial for tailoring an effective metabolic confusion diet plan, especially for endomorphic women aiming to achieve a leaner physique.

Endomorph

Characteristics: Endomorphs typically have a higher percentage of body fat, often distributed around the hips, thighs, and abdomen. They possess a rounder, softer body shape with a wider waist and larger bone structure. This body type tends to have a slower metabolism, making it easier to gain weight but more challenging to lose it.

Metabolic Tendencies: Endomorphs often struggle with insulin sensitivity, meaning their bodies are more likely to convert excess carbohydrates into fat rather than using them for energy. This predisposition necessitates a careful balance of macronutrients, with an emphasis on higher protein and healthy fat intake, and a controlled consumption of carbohydrates.

Nutritional Needs: For endomorphs, a diet rich in lean proteins, healthy fats, and low-glycemic carbohydrates is ideal. This approach helps to stabilize blood sugar levels, enhance satiety, and prevent fat accumulation. Regular physical activity, particularly a mix of resistance training and cardiovascular exercise, is also essential to boost metabolism and promote fat loss.

Mesomorph

Characteristics: Mesomorphs are naturally muscular and possess a more athletic build. They have a medium-sized bone structure, broad shoulders, and a narrow waist. This body type typically has a balanced distribution of muscle and fat, giving them a naturally fit appearance.

Metabolic Tendencies: Mesomorphs usually have a more efficient metabolism, allowing them to gain muscle and lose fat relatively easily. They respond well to both resistance training and aerobic exercises, making them highly adaptable to various fitness routines.

Nutritional Needs: A balanced diet with a moderate intake of carbohydrates, proteins, and fats suits mesomorphs best. They should focus on maintaining their muscle mass through adequate protein intake and supporting their energy needs with complex carbohydrates and healthy fats. Given their natural propensity for muscle gain, mesomorphs should incorporate a variety of exercises to continually challenge their bodies.

Ectomorph

Characteristics: Ectomorphs are characterized by a lean, slender physique with a narrow frame, small joints, and long limbs. They have a low body fat percentage and find it challenging to gain both muscle and fat.

Metabolic Tendencies: Ectomorphs generally have a fast metabolism, which allows them to burn calories quickly. This high metabolic rate makes it difficult for them to gain weight, whether it be muscle or fat. They require a higher caloric intake to meet their energy needs.

Nutritional Needs: Ectomorphs benefit from a diet that is higher in carbohydrates and calories to support their fast metabolism. They should focus on nutrient-dense foods that provide sustained energy and promote muscle growth. Regular strength training is crucial for ectomorphs to build and maintain muscle mass, while cardiovascular exercise should be moderate to avoid excessive calorie expenditure.

Applying This Knowledge

Recognizing these somatotypes allows individuals to tailor their dietary and exercise regimens effectively. For endomorphic women, understanding their unique metabolic challenges and adopting a strategic metabolic confusion diet can help optimize fat loss and muscle gain. By integrating personalized nutrition and fitness plans based on their body type, individuals can achieve their health and weight loss goals more efficiently and sustainably.

Chapter 1: Understanding Your Body Type

In this chapter, we delve into the fundamental concept of body types, or somatotypes, and how they influence your approach to weight loss and fitness. By understanding the distinct characteristics and metabolic tendencies of endomorphs, mesomorphs, and ectomorphs, you can tailor your diet and exercise regimen to suit your unique needs. This knowledge is pivotal for crafting an effective metabolic confusion diet plan, especially designed for endomorphic women. We will explore the physiological traits, metabolic responses, and optimal nutritional strategies for each body type, empowering you with the insights needed to embark on your weight loss journey with confidence and precision.

What is an Endomorph?

In this section, we will explore the endomorph body type, a classification characterized by specific physiological and metabolic traits. Endomorphs typically possess a higher percentage of body fat, a rounder physique, and a predisposition to easily gain weight, especially in the form of fat rather than muscle. This body type often features a slower metabolism, which can make weight loss more challenging compared to other somatotypes.

Understanding the endomorph body type is crucial for tailoring an effective diet and exercise plan. The endomorphic metabolism is less efficient at burning calories, leading to a higher likelihood of fat storage. Consequently, endomorphs may struggle with weight management and require a strategic approach to nutrition and physical activity to achieve their health goals.

By identifying the unique characteristics and needs of endomorphs, this book aims to provide you with the tools and knowledge necessary to optimize your metabolic health. We will delve into the science behind the endomorph body type, discussing how to leverage dietary choices and exercise routines to overcome metabolic hurdles. This foundational understanding will set the stage for implementing the metabolic confusion diet, a dynamic approach designed to keep your metabolism active and responsive.

This section will equip you with the insights needed to navigate the challenges associated with the endomorph body type, empowering you to make informed decisions and adopt sustainable habits for long-term success.

Characteristics and Traits

Understanding the characteristics and traits of the endomorph body type is essential for developing an effective weight management and health optimization strategy. Endomorphs possess distinct physiological and metabolic features that influence their propensity for weight gain and their approach to diet and exercise. Here, we detail the primary characteristics and traits of the endomorph body type:

Body Composition

Endomorphs typically have a higher percentage of body fat compared to ectomorphs and mesomorphs. This fat is often distributed around the abdomen, hips, and thighs, leading to a rounder and softer appearance. While muscle mass can be developed, it is often less prominent due to the higher fat composition.

Metabolic Rate

One of the defining traits of endomorphs is a slower metabolic rate. This means that their bodies are less efficient at burning calories, which can result in a higher tendency to store fat. The reduced metabolic rate makes it crucial for endomorphs to manage their caloric intake carefully and engage in regular physical activity to stimulate their metabolism.

Insulin Sensitivity

Endomorphs often exhibit higher levels of insulin sensitivity, making them more prone to storing carbohydrates as fat. This sensitivity can lead to fluctuations in blood sugar levels and increased fat storage if carbohydrate intake is not properly managed. A diet lower in refined carbohydrates and higher in protein and healthy fats can help mitigate these effects.

Hormonal Influences

Hormonal imbalances can significantly impact the endomorph body type. Higher levels of estrogen and lower levels of testosterone are common, contributing to fat accumulation and making muscle building more challenging. Understanding these hormonal influences is critical for tailoring a diet and exercise program that supports hormonal balance and fat loss.

Physical Traits

Endomorphs typically have a larger bone structure, with wider hips and shoulders. They may also have shorter limbs and a more compact body shape. These physical traits can influence their exercise capabilities and preferences, making certain types of physical activity more suitable and effective than others.

Dietary Response

Due to their metabolic characteristics, endomorphs often respond better to diets that are higher in protein and healthy fats while being lower in carbohydrates. This dietary approach can help stabilize blood sugar levels, reduce cravings, and promote fat loss. Endomorphs benefit from nutrient-dense, whole foods that provide sustained energy and support metabolic health.

Exercise Preferences

Endomorphs tend to excel in strength-based and endurance activities rather than high-intensity, explosive exercises. Incorporating a mix of cardio, strength training, and flexibility exercises can help endomorphs optimize their fitness routine, improve muscle mass, and enhance metabolic rate.

By recognizing and understanding these characteristics and traits, endomorphs can adopt more effective strategies for weight management and overall health. This foundational knowledge will guide the development of personalized dietary and exercise plans that cater to the unique needs of the endomorph body type, facilitating more sustainable and successful health outcomes.

Common Challenges Faced by Endomorphs

Endomorphs face unique challenges related to their body composition, metabolic rate, and overall health. Understanding these challenges is crucial for developing effective strategies to manage weight and improve well-being. This section delves into the common challenges faced by endomorphs and offers insights into addressing these issues.

1. Weight Gain and Difficulty Losing Weight

One of the most significant challenges for endomorphs is their propensity to gain weight easily. This is primarily due to their slower metabolic rate, which means their bodies burn calories more slowly than those of ectomorphs and mesomorphs. As a result, endomorphs often struggle with weight gain even when consuming a relatively modest number of calories. Losing weight can be equally challenging because creating a calorie deficit often requires more effort and discipline.

2. High Body Fat Percentage

Endomorphs typically have a higher body fat percentage, particularly around the midsection, hips, and thighs. This distribution of body fat can increase the risk of developing conditions such as metabolic syndrome, type 2 diabetes, and cardiovascular disease. The higher body fat percentage also impacts physical appearance and can be a source of frustration and self-consciousness.

3. Insulin Resistance and Blood Sugar Fluctuations

Endomorphs are often more prone to insulin resistance, a condition where the body's cells do not respond effectively to insulin. This can lead to elevated blood sugar levels and increased fat storage, particularly after consuming carbohydrates. Managing insulin resistance typically involves careful monitoring of carbohydrate intake and prioritizing foods that help stabilize blood sugar levels.

4. Hormonal Imbalances

Hormonal imbalances are another common challenge for endomorphs. They often have higher levels of estrogen and lower levels of testosterone, which can contribute to increased fat storage and difficulty building muscle mass. Hormonal imbalances can also affect energy levels, mood, and overall metabolic health, making it essential to adopt lifestyle practices that promote hormonal balance.

5. Low Energy Levels and Fatigue

Due to their slower metabolism and higher body fat percentage, endomorphs may experience lower energy levels and fatigue more frequently than other body types. This can impact their ability to engage in regular physical activity, further exacerbating weight management challenges. Addressing fatigue often requires a comprehensive approach, including a balanced diet, regular exercise, and adequate sleep.

6. Cravings and Appetite Control

Endomorphs often struggle with cravings, particularly for high-carbohydrate and sugary foods. These cravings can lead to overeating and difficulty sticking to a healthy eating plan. Managing cravings and appetite control typically involves consuming a diet rich in protein, healthy fats, and fiber, which helps promote satiety and reduce the urge to snack on unhealthy foods.

7. Psychological and Emotional Challenges

The physical challenges faced by endomorphs can also have psychological and emotional repercussions. Feelings of frustration, low self-esteem, and body image issues are common among endomorphs who struggle with their weight. These psychological challenges can impact motivation and adherence to a healthy lifestyle. Support from healthcare professionals, counselors, and support groups can be beneficial in addressing these emotional aspects.

8. Limited Exercise Tolerance

Due to their body composition, endomorphs may find certain types of exercise more challenging. High-impact or high-intensity workouts can be difficult to sustain, leading to discouragement and reduced physical activity levels. Finding the right balance of cardio, strength training, and low-impact exercises is crucial for maintaining an effective and enjoyable fitness routine.

By understanding and addressing these common challenges, endomorphs can develop more effective strategies for managing their weight and improving their overall health. The key is to adopt a holistic approach that combines dietary modifications, regular physical activity, and lifestyle changes tailored to the unique needs of the endomorph body type.

What is a Mesomorph?

Mesomorphs represent one of the three primary somatotypes and are often considered the most naturally athletic body type. Characterized by a well-proportioned physique, mesomorphs typically exhibit a high degree of muscularity and a low-to-moderate amount of body fat. This body type is naturally predisposed to muscle growth and strength, making it advantageous for both athletic performance and physical aesthetics.

Individuals with a mesomorphic body type often find it easier to gain muscle and maintain a lean body composition compared to endomorphs and ectomorphs. This ease of muscle gain and fat loss is primarily due to their more efficient metabolism and favorable hormonal profile, which supports anabolic (muscle-building) processes. As a result, mesomorphs are generally more responsive to both resistance training and cardiovascular exercise, allowing for a versatile and adaptable approach to fitness.

Mesomorphs tend to have broad shoulders, a narrow waist, and a naturally strong and muscular build. This body type often excels in activities that require strength, power, and agility, making it ideal for a wide range of sports and physical pursuits. Additionally, mesomorphs usually have a higher resting metabolic rate, which contributes to their ability to burn calories efficiently and maintain a healthy weight.

Despite these advantages, mesomorphs must still adhere to a balanced diet and consistent exercise regimen to maximize their genetic potential and avoid potential pitfalls such as overtraining or nutritional imbalances. Understanding the unique characteristics and needs of the mesomorphic body type is essential for optimizing health, performance, and overall well-being. In the following sections, we will explore the specific traits, challenges, and strategies associated with this somatotype, providing a comprehensive guide for mesomorphs looking to achieve their fitness goals.

Characteristics and Traits

The mesomorph body type is often recognized for its distinct physical attributes and advantageous physiological traits. This somatotype is naturally predisposed to muscularity, making it an ideal body type for both aesthetic and athletic pursuits. Here, we delve into the key characteristics and traits that define mesomorphs.

Physical Characteristics

1. **Muscular Build:** Mesomorphs are characterized by a naturally muscular physique. They tend to develop muscle mass easily and have a more defined and prominent musculature compared to endomorphs and ectomorphs. This muscular build is often apparent even without extensive training.

2. **Proportional Body:** Individuals with a mesomorphic body type typically have well-proportioned bodies. They possess broad shoulders and a narrow waist, which contributes to an aesthetically pleasing V-shaped torso. This proportionality enhances their physical appearance and performance in various sports.

3. **Bone Structure:** Mesomorphs have a medium to large bone structure. This robust skeletal frame provides a solid foundation for muscle attachment and growth, further enhancing their strength and power capabilities.

4. **Body Fat Distribution:** Mesomorphs generally have a lower body fat percentage. When they do gain fat, it is often evenly distributed, which helps in maintaining a balanced and symmetrical physique.

5. **Height and Weight:** While mesomorphs can vary in height, they often exhibit a balance between muscle mass and body weight. This balance contributes to their overall physical agility and capability.

Metabolic Traits

1. **Efficient Metabolism:** Mesomorphs typically have a higher basal metabolic rate (BMR), which means they burn calories more efficiently at rest. This metabolic efficiency aids in maintaining a lean physique and supports muscle growth and recovery.

2. **Hormonal Profile:** The hormonal environment of mesomorphs is often conducive to muscle building and fat loss. They tend to have higher levels of anabolic hormones such as testosterone and growth hormone, which promote muscle protein synthesis and overall physical development.

3. **Adaptability to Exercise:** Mesomorphs respond exceptionally well to both resistance training and cardiovascular exercise. Their bodies adapt quickly to physical activity, allowing for rapid gains in strength, endurance, and muscle hypertrophy.

Behavioral and Psychological Traits

1. **High Physical Activity Levels:** Mesomorphs are often naturally inclined towards physical activity. They enjoy and excel in sports and fitness-related pursuits, which further reinforces their muscular and athletic build.

2. **Motivation and Drive:** Due to their natural physical advantages, mesomorphs often have a strong motivation to engage in regular exercise and maintain an active lifestyle. This intrinsic drive helps them achieve and sustain their fitness goals.

3. **Body Image Confidence:** The favorable physical characteristics of mesomorphs often lead to higher levels of body confidence and self-esteem. This positive body image can be a motivating factor in adhering to healthy lifestyle choices.

Understanding these characteristics and traits is crucial for tailoring fitness and nutrition strategies that optimize the mesomorphic potential. By recognizing and leveraging their natural advantages, mesomorphs can achieve remarkable results in both physical performance and overall health. In the following sections, we will explore the common challenges faced by mesomorphs and effective strategies to overcome them.

Benefits of Transitioning to a Mesomorph Body Type

Transitioning to a mesomorph body type, while not entirely possible due to genetic predispositions, can still be a goal for many individuals looking to improve their physical health and appearance. By adopting certain lifestyle changes, dietary adjustments, and targeted exercise routines, one can harness the benefits commonly associated with the mesomorphic body type. Here, we delve into the specific advantages of aiming for and achieving a physique closer to that of a mesomorph.

Enhanced Muscle Mass and Strength

1. **Increased Muscle Hypertrophy:** One of the primary benefits of transitioning towards a mesomorphic body type is the potential for increased muscle mass. Mesomorphs naturally gain muscle more easily due to their genetic makeup, and by adopting similar training regimens, individuals can enhance muscle hypertrophy, leading to a more muscular and defined physique.

2. **Improved Strength and Power:** With increased muscle mass comes greater strength and power. This enhancement is beneficial not only for athletic performance but also for everyday functional activities, reducing the risk of injury and improving overall quality of life.

Optimal Metabolic Function

1. **Higher Basal Metabolic Rate (BMR):** Mesomorphs typically have a higher BMR, meaning they burn more calories at rest. By increasing muscle mass through resistance training and adequate nutrition, individuals can boost their metabolic rate, facilitating easier weight management and fat loss.

2. **Efficient Energy Utilization:** Enhanced muscle mass contributes to better energy utilization. Muscles are metabolically active tissues that require energy for maintenance and function, leading to improved overall energy levels and stamina.

Aesthetic and Physical Appeal

1. **Proportional and Balanced Physique:** Achieving a physique that resembles the mesomorph body type often results in a well-proportioned and balanced appearance. Broad shoulders, a narrow waist, and a defined musculature contribute to the classic V-shaped torso that is widely considered aesthetically pleasing.
2. **Reduced Body Fat:** Transitioning towards a mesomorphic physique typically involves a reduction in body fat percentage. This not only enhances physical appearance but also contributes to better health outcomes by reducing the risk of obesity-related conditions.

Psychological and Behavioral Benefits

1. **Increased Self-Confidence:** Improvements in physical appearance and strength often lead to increased self-confidence and self-esteem. This positive body image can enhance mental health and overall well-being.
2. **Motivation for Active Lifestyle:** The visible results from training and dietary efforts can serve as powerful motivation to maintain an active and healthy lifestyle. This ongoing commitment to fitness and health can lead to sustained improvements in physical and mental health.

Health Advantages

1. **Reduced Risk of Chronic Diseases:** Lower body fat percentages and increased muscle mass are associated with a reduced risk of chronic diseases such as cardiovascular disease, type 2 diabetes, and certain cancers. By aiming for a mesomorphic physique, individuals can improve their overall health profile.
2. **Enhanced Bone Health:** Resistance training, a key component of transitioning towards a mesomorphic body type, is known to improve bone density and strength. This is particularly beneficial in reducing the risk of osteoporosis and fractures.

Improved Athletic Performance

1. **Better Physical Performance:** The strength, power, and endurance gains associated with increased muscle mass can significantly improve athletic performance. This is beneficial for both competitive athletes and recreational exercisers.
2. **Injury Prevention:** A stronger musculoskeletal system, resulting from resistance training and increased muscle mass, can help prevent injuries. Enhanced stability and support around joints reduce the likelihood of strains, sprains, and other common injuries.

What is an Ectomorph?

An ectomorph is one of the three primary body types, or somatotypes, first described by psychologist William H. Sheldon in the 1940s. Ectomorphs are characterized by their slender, lean physique, often featuring long limbs, narrow shoulders, and minimal body fat and muscle mass. This body type is genetically predisposed to a fast metabolism, which makes gaining weight and muscle mass more challenging compared to mesomorphs and endomorphs. Understanding the ectomorphic body type is crucial for tailoring specific fitness and nutritional strategies that align with its unique physiological characteristics.

Individuals with an ectomorphic body type typically have a high metabolic rate, which means their bodies burn calories more rapidly. This rapid metabolism, while advantageous for maintaining a lean physique, can pose challenges in muscle and weight gain. Ectomorphs often struggle to consume enough calories to meet their body's energy demands, especially when engaging in intense physical activities or strength training.

Recognizing the specific traits and challenges of the ectomorphic body type is essential for developing effective fitness and dietary plans. Strategies often include increased caloric intake, focusing on nutrient-dense foods, and incorporating resistance training to promote muscle hypertrophy. Ectomorphs may benefit from a diet rich in proteins and complex carbohydrates to support their high energy expenditure and muscle-building efforts.

In this subchapter, we will delve deeper into the characteristics and traits of ectomorphs, explore the common challenges they face, and provide practical guidance on how to optimize health and fitness outcomes for this body type. Understanding these nuances can empower ectomorphs to achieve their health and fitness goals more effectively.

Characteristics and Traits

Ectomorphs exhibit a distinctive set of physical characteristics and metabolic traits that differentiate them from endomorphs and mesomorphs. Understanding these unique features is crucial for developing effective fitness and nutritional strategies tailored to this body type.

Physical Characteristics

1. **Slender Build**: Ectomorphs typically have a naturally thin and lean physique. They possess narrow shoulders, chest, and hips, giving them a delicate frame.

2. **Long Limbs**: One of the most noticeable traits of ectomorphs is their long arms and legs. This elongation contributes to their overall slender appearance and often makes them excel in activities that benefit from a greater reach, such as swimming or basketball.

3. **Low Body Fat**: Ectomorphs generally have low levels of body fat. Their bodies are efficient at burning calories, which makes it difficult for them to gain and maintain body fat. This trait contributes to their naturally lean and often wiry look.

4. **Small Joints and Bones**: Ectomorphs usually have small joints and bones, which further accentuates their slim build. Their wrists and ankles are often noticeably thin compared to those of mesomorphs or endomorphs.

Metabolic Traits

1. **High Metabolic Rate**: A defining characteristic of ectomorphs is their fast metabolism. They tend to burn calories quickly, which can be advantageous for maintaining a lean physique but challenging when trying to gain weight or muscle mass.

2. **Difficulty Gaining Weight**: Due to their high metabolic rate, ectomorphs often struggle to gain weight. This includes both muscle mass and body fat. Even with increased caloric intake, their bodies tend to burn off the excess calories efficiently.

3. **High Energy Levels**: Ectomorphs often have high energy levels, which can be attributed to their fast metabolism. This trait makes them well-suited for endurance activities and sports that require sustained energy over long periods.

4. **Rapid Recovery**: Ectomorphs generally experience quick recovery times after physical activities. Their bodies are adept at processing and utilizing nutrients efficiently, which aids in faster recuperation from workouts and other physical exertions.

Behavioral and Lifestyle Traits

1. **Active Lifestyle**: Many ectomorphs naturally gravitate towards an active lifestyle due to their high energy levels. They are often engaged in various physical activities and sports, which helps them stay fit and lean.

2. **High Caloric Needs**: To support their fast metabolism and active lifestyle, ectomorphs require a higher caloric intake compared to endomorphs and mesomorphs. This need can make it challenging to consume enough food, especially nutrient-dense options, to meet their energy demands.
3. **Preference for Carbohydrates**: Ectomorphs often have a preference for carbohydrate-rich foods. Their bodies utilize carbohydrates efficiently for energy, which can lead to cravings for foods high in carbs.

Understanding these characteristics and traits is essential for ectomorphs to tailor their diet and exercise plans effectively. By recognizing their unique metabolic and physical attributes, ectomorphs can develop strategies that help them achieve their health and fitness goals, whether it's gaining muscle mass, maintaining a lean physique, or enhancing overall well-being.

Benefits of Transitioning to an Ectomorph Body Type

Transitioning to an ectomorph body type, while inherently challenging due to genetic and metabolic predispositions, offers numerous benefits for overall health and well-being. Understanding these benefits can provide motivation and clarity for individuals aiming to adopt characteristics typical of an ectomorphic physique.

Enhanced Metabolic Efficiency

1. **Increased Caloric Expenditure**: Ectomorphs typically have a higher basal metabolic rate (BMR), which means their bodies burn more calories at rest. This enhanced caloric expenditure can aid in maintaining a lean body composition, making it easier to manage body weight and prevent obesity-related health issues.
2. **Improved Insulin Sensitivity**: Higher metabolic rates are often associated with better insulin sensitivity. This means the body is more efficient at managing blood sugar levels, reducing the risk of developing insulin resistance and type 2 diabetes.

Cardiovascular Health

1. **Lower Risk of Cardiovascular Disease**: A leaner body composition with lower levels of body fat, common among ectomorphs, is linked to a reduced risk of cardiovascular diseases. Maintaining a healthy weight can decrease blood pressure, improve lipid profiles, and enhance overall heart health.
2. **Enhanced Endurance**: Ectomorphs often excel in endurance activities due to their efficient energy metabolism and lighter body weight. This can lead to improved cardiovascular endurance, enabling longer and more effective aerobic workouts, which are crucial for heart health.

Musculoskeletal Benefits

1. **Reduced Joint Stress**: Carrying less body weight reduces the stress on joints, particularly in weight-bearing activities. This can lower the risk of developing joint-related issues such as osteoarthritis, enhancing overall mobility and physical activity levels.
2. **Improved Flexibility and Agility**: Ectomorphs often possess a natural agility and flexibility due to their lighter and leaner build. This can enhance performance in various physical activities and sports, reducing the risk of injuries.

Psychological and Lifestyle Advantages

1. **Body Image and Self-Esteem**: Achieving and maintaining a lean physique can significantly improve body image and self-esteem. The societal perception of a lean body as being healthy and fit can boost confidence and psychological well-being.
2. **Sustained Energy Levels**: The high metabolic rate of ectomorphs contributes to sustained energy levels throughout the day. This can improve productivity, enhance mood, and support a more active and engaged lifestyle.

Disease Prevention

1. **Lower Risk of Metabolic Syndrome**: A lean body composition with low levels of visceral fat can significantly reduce the risk of metabolic syndrome, a cluster of conditions that increase the risk of heart disease, stroke, and diabetes.
2. **Cancer Risk Reduction**: Research suggests that lower body fat percentages are associated with a reduced risk of certain types of cancers, including breast and colorectal cancers. Maintaining a lean physique can be a preventive measure against these and other cancers.

Longevity and Quality of Life

1. **Increased Longevity**: Numerous studies have indicated that maintaining a lean body composition is linked to increased life expectancy. Lower levels of body fat can reduce the risk of chronic diseases, contributing to a longer and healthier life.
2. **Enhanced Quality of Life**: The combination of physical health, psychological well-being, and reduced disease risk leads to an overall enhanced quality of life. Individuals can enjoy more active, fulfilling lives with fewer health-related limitations.

Practical Considerations

1. **Simplified Weight Management**: Once an ectomorphic state is achieved, managing weight becomes more straightforward due to the body's efficient calorie-burning capabilities. This simplifies dietary planning and reduces the need for extreme dietary restrictions.
2. **Varied Diet and Flexibility**: Ectomorphs can often enjoy a more varied diet with higher caloric intake without significant weight gain. This flexibility can make it easier to maintain a balanced and nutritious diet.

While the transition to an ectomorphic body type requires dedication and strategic planning, the benefits span numerous aspects of health and well-being. By understanding and leveraging these advantages, individuals can achieve a healthier, more active lifestyle and improve their overall quality of life.

The Science Behind Metabolism

Metabolism is a fundamental biological process that governs how our bodies convert food into energy. Understanding the science behind metabolism is crucial for anyone looking to manage their weight and improve their overall health. Metabolism encompasses all the chemical reactions that occur within our cells, providing the energy necessary for vital functions such as breathing, digestion, and physical activity. It is divided into two main categories: catabolism, which breaks down molecules to release energy, and anabolism, which uses energy to construct components of cells such as proteins and nucleic acids.

The rate at which your body burns calories, known as your metabolic rate, is influenced by several factors, including genetics, age, sex, body composition, and physical activity level. Basal metabolic rate (BMR) is the amount of energy expended while at rest in a neutrally temperate environment, and it accounts for the largest portion of your total daily energy expenditure. Other factors, such as thermogenesis (the process of heat production in organisms) and physical activity, also play significant roles.

Hormones, particularly those produced by the thyroid gland, significantly impact metabolic rate. Thyroxine (T4) and triiodothyronine (T3) are key hormones that regulate metabolism. Additionally, insulin and glucagon from the pancreas help manage glucose levels, influencing energy storage and usage.

Understanding the intricacies of metabolism provides insight into how dietary choices, exercise, and lifestyle habits can be optimized to support weight loss and overall health. This knowledge forms the foundation for effectively implementing dietary strategies such as the metabolic confusion diet, which aims to harness the body's natural metabolic processes to facilitate weight management and health improvement.

Metabolic Rates and Hormonal Influence

Metabolic rate refers to the speed at which the body converts food into energy. This rate varies significantly among individuals and is influenced by a multitude of factors, including age, sex, body composition, genetic predisposition, and physical activity levels. Understanding metabolic rates and the hormonal influences on metabolism is essential for optimizing dietary and exercise interventions to enhance weight management and overall health.

Basal Metabolic Rate (BMR)

The Basal Metabolic Rate (BMR) represents the amount of energy expended by the body at rest to maintain vital physiological functions, such as breathing, circulation, cell production, nutrient processing, and temperature regulation. BMR accounts for approximately 60-75% of total daily energy expenditure in sedentary individuals. Factors influencing BMR include:

1. **Age**: BMR decreases with age due to loss of lean muscle mass and hormonal changes.

2. **Sex**: Men typically have a higher BMR than women, primarily due to greater muscle mass.

3. **Body Composition**: Muscle tissue burns more calories at rest compared to fat tissue, thus individuals with higher muscle mass have a higher BMR.

4. **Genetics**: Genetic predisposition can influence metabolic efficiency and BMR.

Hormonal Regulation

Hormones play a pivotal role in regulating metabolism. Key hormones involved include:

1. **Thyroid Hormones (T3 and T4)**: Produced by the thyroid gland, thyroxine (T4) and triiodothyronine (T3) significantly influence metabolic rate. T3 is the more active form, increasing the rate of cellular metabolism. Hypothyroidism (low thyroid hormone levels) can lead to a reduced metabolic rate, weight gain, and fatigue, whereas hyperthyroidism (high thyroid hormone levels) can increase metabolic rate, causing weight loss and increased energy expenditure.

2. **Insulin**: Produced by the pancreas, insulin regulates glucose uptake by cells and influences fat storage. Insulin resistance, a condition where cells fail to respond effectively to insulin, can lead to impaired glucose metabolism and is associated with obesity and metabolic syndrome.

3. **Glucagon**: Also produced by the pancreas, glucagon works antagonistically to insulin by promoting the release of stored glucose from the liver, thereby increasing blood glucose levels. This hormone helps maintain energy balance during fasting and exercise.

4. **Cortisol**: Known as the stress hormone, cortisol is produced by the adrenal glands. It plays a role in energy regulation by increasing blood sugar through gluconeogenesis and promoting the breakdown of muscle protein. Chronic high levels of cortisol can lead to increased appetite and fat deposition, particularly in the abdominal area.

5. **Leptin and Ghrelin**: Leptin, produced by adipose tissue, signals satiety and helps regulate energy balance by inhibiting hunger. Ghrelin, produced in the stomach, stimulates appetite. Imbalances in these hormones can lead to dysregulated appetite control and weight gain.

Adaptive Thermogenesis

Adaptive thermogenesis is the process by which the body adjusts its energy expenditure in response to changes in diet and physical activity. This mechanism is influenced by hormonal signals and can alter the efficiency of calorie utilization. For example, during prolonged caloric restriction, the body may lower its metabolic rate to conserve energy, making weight loss more challenging.

Understanding these complex interactions between metabolic rates and hormonal influences is crucial for designing effective weight management strategies. By leveraging this knowledge, individuals can tailor their dietary and exercise plans to align with their unique metabolic profiles, thereby optimizing health outcomes and achieving sustainable weight loss.

How Metabolic Confusion Works

Metabolic confusion, also known as calorie cycling or calorie shifting, is an innovative dietary approach designed to prevent the body from adapting to a consistent caloric intake. This method aims to "confuse" the metabolism by varying the number of calories consumed on different days or weeks, thereby enhancing metabolic rate and promoting weight loss. Understanding how metabolic confusion works requires a detailed examination of its physiological and biochemical mechanisms.

The Principle of Metabolic Adaptation

The human body is highly adaptive and strives to maintain homeostasis. When subjected to a prolonged caloric deficit, the body adjusts by lowering its Basal Metabolic Rate (BMR) to conserve energy. This adaptive thermogenesis can lead to a plateau in weight loss, as the body becomes more efficient at functioning with fewer calories. Metabolic confusion seeks to counteract this adaptive response by periodically increasing caloric intake, preventing the metabolic rate from dropping significantly.

Mechanisms of Metabolic Confusion

1. **Preventing Adaptive Thermogenesis**

    - **Caloric Cycling**: By alternating between high-calorie and low-calorie days, the body is unable to predict and adapt to a consistent caloric intake. This prevents the metabolic rate from decreasing, as the body does not enter a prolonged state of perceived caloric deprivation.

    - **Thermogenic Effect of Food**: Varying caloric intake influences the thermogenic effect of food, which is the energy required for digestion, absorption, and metabolism of nutrients. Higher calorie days may enhance this thermogenic effect, thereby increasing overall energy expenditure.

2. **Hormonal Regulation**

    - **Leptin and Ghrelin**: Metabolic confusion can help regulate the hormones leptin and ghrelin, which control hunger and satiety. Higher calorie days can boost leptin levels, reducing hunger and increasing feelings of fullness, while preventing the chronic elevation of ghrelin that typically accompanies prolonged caloric restriction.

    - **Insulin Sensitivity**: Fluctuating caloric intake can improve insulin sensitivity. High-calorie days with controlled macronutrient distribution can prevent insulin resistance, a common issue in consistent low-calorie diets.

3. **Maintaining Muscle Mass**
    - **Protein Intake**: During low-calorie phases, adequate protein intake is crucial to prevent muscle catabolism. High-calorie days allow for increased protein consumption, which supports muscle maintenance and growth, thus preserving lean body mass and sustaining a higher metabolic rate.
    - **Muscle Protein Synthesis**: Increased caloric intake on certain days provides the necessary substrates for muscle protein synthesis, preventing the loss of muscle mass that can occur with continuous low-calorie diets.
4. **Psychological Benefits**
    - **Diet Adherence**: The flexibility of metabolic confusion can improve adherence to dietary regimens. Knowing that higher calorie days are part of the plan can reduce feelings of deprivation and the psychological strain associated with constant caloric restriction.
    - **Reduced Binge Eating**: By incorporating regular high-calorie days, the likelihood of uncontrolled binge eating episodes may decrease. This structured approach to periodic increased caloric intake can help manage cravings and maintain consistent dietary habits.

Practical Implementation

Implementing metabolic confusion involves strategically planning caloric intake:

- **High-Calorie Days**: These days involve consuming calories at or slightly above maintenance level, typically ranging from 2000-2500 calories for women, depending on individual factors such as age, activity level, and metabolic rate.
- **Low-Calorie Days**: These days involve a caloric deficit, generally around 1200-1500 calories, to promote weight loss while ensuring adequate nutrient intake to prevent muscle loss and nutrient deficiencies.
- **Macronutrient Distribution**: Ensuring a balanced intake of macronutrients (proteins, fats, and carbohydrates) tailored to individual metabolic needs on both high and low-calorie days.

Evidence and Efficacy

Research on metabolic confusion has shown promising results in enhancing weight loss and maintaining metabolic rate. Studies indicate that alternating caloric intake can result in greater fat loss, improved insulin sensitivity, and higher diet adherence compared to continuous caloric restriction. However, more extensive, long-term studies are needed to fully understand the benefits and optimize protocols for different populations.

Chapter 2: The Metabolic Confusion Diet

The Metabolic Confusion Diet represents a dynamic and adaptive approach to weight management, particularly effective for individuals with an endomorphic body type. This chapter delves into the principles and practical applications of metabolic confusion, explaining how alternating between high-calorie and low-calorie intake can optimize metabolic function and facilitate weight loss. By preventing metabolic adaptation and promoting hormonal balance, this dietary strategy offers a sustainable and flexible pathway to achieving your health goals. Here, we will explore detailed guidelines, meal plans, and scientific evidence supporting the effectiveness of the Metabolic Confusion Diet.

Introduction to Metabolic Confusion

Metabolic confusion, also known as calorie cycling or calorie shifting, is an innovative dietary approach designed to optimize metabolic function and enhance weight management. Unlike traditional diets that impose a consistent calorie restriction, metabolic confusion involves alternating between periods of higher and lower caloric intake. This strategic variation aims to "confuse" the body's metabolic processes, preventing the adaptive thermogenesis that often leads to weight loss plateaus.

The core principle of metabolic confusion lies in its ability to maintain metabolic rate and hormonal balance. By varying calorie intake, the body is less likely to enter a state of metabolic slowdown, which is a common response to prolonged caloric restriction. This approach leverages the body's natural adaptability, encouraging it to continue burning calories efficiently even as dietary intake fluctuates.

In this subchapter, we will explore the scientific foundations of metabolic confusion, examining how it influences metabolic rates and hormonal responses. We will also discuss the practical aspects of implementing this diet, including how to structure high and low-calorie days effectively. Understanding these principles is crucial for maximizing the benefits of metabolic confusion and achieving sustainable weight loss.

Furthermore, metabolic confusion is particularly beneficial for endomorphs, who typically face challenges such as slower metabolism and easier fat accumulation. By adopting this flexible dietary strategy, individuals can overcome these hurdles, promoting a healthier body composition and improved overall well-being. As we delve into the details, you will gain insights into how to tailor this approach to fit your lifestyle and dietary preferences, setting the stage for long-term success.

Definition and Principles

Definition of Metabolic Confusion

Metabolic confusion, also referred to as calorie cycling or calorie shifting, is a dietary strategy that alternates between periods of high and low caloric intake to prevent the body from adapting to a consistent calorie deficit. This approach is designed to keep the metabolism "guessing," thereby maintaining a higher metabolic rate and promoting sustained weight loss. Unlike traditional diets that involve continuous calorie restriction, metabolic confusion introduces variability in daily caloric intake, which can help mitigate the body's natural tendency to slow down its metabolic processes in response to prolonged dieting.

Principles of Metabolic Confusion

1. **Alternating Caloric Intake:** The fundamental principle of metabolic confusion is the strategic alternation between high-calorie and low-calorie days. High-calorie days involve consuming calories at or above maintenance levels, while low-calorie days involve a significant reduction in caloric intake. This variation helps to prevent the metabolic slowdown that typically accompanies continuous calorie restriction.

2. **Preventing Metabolic Adaptation:** When the body is subjected to a consistent calorie deficit, it adapts by reducing its metabolic rate to conserve energy, a process known as adaptive thermogenesis. By alternating caloric intake, metabolic confusion aims to prevent this adaptation, keeping the metabolism more active and responsive to energy expenditure.

3. **Enhancing Hormonal Balance:** Hormones play a critical role in regulating metabolism and appetite. Continuous calorie restriction can lead to hormonal imbalances, such as reduced levels of leptin (which signals satiety) and increased levels of ghrelin (which stimulates hunger). By varying caloric intake, metabolic confusion helps to maintain a more balanced hormonal environment, reducing hunger and promoting satiety.

4. **Flexibility and Sustainability:** One of the key advantages of metabolic confusion is its flexibility. This approach allows individuals to enjoy periods of higher caloric intake, which can make the diet more sustainable over the long term. The ability to incorporate higher-calorie days can also improve adherence to the diet, as it reduces the psychological burden of constant restriction.

5. **Customization and Personalization:** Metabolic confusion can be tailored to individual needs and preferences. The frequency and magnitude of caloric shifts can be adjusted based on factors such as activity level, metabolic rate, and weight loss goals. This customization ensures that the diet is both effective and manageable for different individuals.

6. **Integration with Exercise:** Regular physical activity is an important component of the metabolic confusion approach. Exercise, particularly strength training, helps to preserve lean muscle mass, which is crucial for maintaining a higher metabolic rate. On high-calorie days, individuals can engage in more intense workouts to take advantage of the increased energy availability.

Implementing Metabolic Confusion

To effectively implement metabolic confusion, individuals should plan their high and low-calorie days in advance. A common approach is to alternate every other day, or to follow a pattern such as five low-calorie days followed by two high-calorie days each week. It is essential to ensure that even on low-calorie days, the diet remains nutritionally balanced, providing adequate protein, healthy fats, and micronutrients.

In conclusion, metabolic confusion offers a dynamic and flexible approach to weight management that leverages the body's natural metabolic processes. By understanding and applying the principles of this diet, individuals can achieve more sustainable weight loss and improved metabolic health.

Benefits of Metabolic Confusion for Endomorphs

Introduction

Endomorphs, characterized by a higher propensity for fat storage and a slower metabolic rate, often face significant challenges in weight management. The metabolic confusion diet offers a strategic approach that can address these unique physiological characteristics. By alternating caloric intake, this diet can provide several benefits specifically tailored to the needs of endomorphs, enhancing their metabolic efficiency and promoting sustainable weight loss.

Enhanced Metabolic Rate

One of the primary benefits of metabolic confusion for endomorphs is the potential to enhance their metabolic rate. Endomorphs typically have a slower metabolism, which can make weight loss more difficult. By incorporating high-calorie days, the metabolic confusion diet helps to prevent the metabolic slowdown that often accompanies continuous calorie restriction. This approach keeps the metabolism more active and responsive, thereby increasing the overall rate of calorie burning and improving weight loss outcomes.

Improved Hormonal Balance

Endomorphs often experience hormonal imbalances that can hinder weight loss efforts. Continuous calorie restriction can exacerbate these issues by reducing levels of leptin, the hormone responsible for signaling satiety, and increasing levels of ghrelin, which stimulates hunger. The metabolic confusion diet, with its alternating high and low-calorie days, helps to maintain a more balanced hormonal environment. This balance reduces hunger and cravings, making it easier for endomorphs to adhere to their dietary plans.

Preservation of Lean Muscle Mass

Maintaining lean muscle mass is crucial for endomorphs, as muscle tissue burns more calories at rest compared to fat tissue. The metabolic confusion diet encourages the preservation of lean muscle mass by integrating periods of higher caloric intake. During these high-calorie days, endomorphs can focus on strength training and other muscle-building activities, ensuring that muscle mass is preserved or even enhanced. This preservation of muscle mass contributes to a higher resting metabolic rate, further aiding in weight management.

Reduction in Psychological Fatigue

Traditional diets that require continuous calorie restriction can lead to psychological fatigue and diet burnout. This is particularly challenging for endomorphs who may already struggle with slower progress in their weight loss journey. The metabolic confusion diet provides periods of higher caloric intake, offering psychological relief and reducing the sense of deprivation. This flexibility makes the diet more sustainable in the long term, as endomorphs are less likely to experience the mental fatigue that often leads to diet abandonment.

Flexibility and Customization

The metabolic confusion diet offers a high degree of flexibility, which is beneficial for endomorphs who may need to adapt their dietary plans to fit their individual needs and lifestyles. The frequency and magnitude of caloric shifts can be customized based on personal preferences, activity levels, and specific weight loss goals. This customization ensures that endomorphs can create a diet plan that is both effective and manageable, increasing the likelihood of long-term success.

Improved Adherence to Exercise Regimens

Endomorphs can benefit from the metabolic confusion diet's encouragement of regular physical activity. High-calorie days provide the energy necessary for more intense workouts, which can include both cardiovascular exercises and strength training. This integration of exercise helps to maximize calorie burn and improve overall fitness levels. The structured variation in caloric intake also helps endomorphs to better align their dietary and exercise efforts, leading to more consistent and effective weight management.

Enhanced Fat Loss

By preventing metabolic adaptation and maintaining a higher metabolic rate, the metabolic confusion diet can lead to enhanced fat loss for endomorphs. The alternating high and low-calorie days create a dynamic energy balance that promotes the efficient use of stored fat as an energy source. This targeted fat loss is particularly beneficial for endomorphs, who tend to store fat more readily, especially in the abdominal region.

Calorie Cycling Explained

Calorie cycling, also known as calorie shifting or metabolic confusion, is an innovative dietary strategy designed to optimize metabolic function and enhance weight loss. Unlike traditional diets that enforce a consistent caloric intake every day, calorie cycling involves alternating between high and low-calorie days. This approach aims to prevent the body's metabolic rate from adapting to a fixed caloric intake, thereby maintaining a higher metabolic rate and promoting efficient fat burning.

The concept behind calorie cycling is grounded in the understanding of metabolic adaptation. When individuals follow a continuous calorie-restricted diet, their metabolism often slows down as the body adapts to conserve energy. This adaptive response can hinder weight loss progress and make it increasingly difficult to shed excess pounds. By varying daily caloric intake, calorie cycling seeks to disrupt this adaptive mechanism, keeping the metabolism active and responsive.

In practice, calorie cycling can be tailored to fit individual needs and lifestyles. For example, one might alternate between days of higher caloric intake, which support intense physical activity and muscle repair, and days of lower caloric intake, which promote fat burning. This flexibility allows for a more sustainable approach to dieting, reducing feelings of deprivation and enhancing adherence to the diet over the long term.

For endomorphs, who typically have slower metabolisms and a higher propensity for fat storage, calorie cycling offers a targeted method to overcome these physiological challenges. By strategically varying caloric intake, endomorphs can stimulate their metabolism, support lean muscle preservation, and achieve more consistent and sustainable weight loss results. This subchapter will delve into the principles and methodologies of calorie cycling, providing a comprehensive understanding of how to effectively implement this approach for optimal metabolic health.

High-Calorie vs. Low-Calorie Days

Calorie cycling involves strategically alternating between high-calorie and low-calorie days to optimize metabolic function and promote weight loss. This approach leverages the body's natural adaptive mechanisms to prevent metabolic slowdown and support sustained fat loss.

High-Calorie Days

High-calorie days are designed to provide the body with an abundance of nutrients and energy, supporting intense physical activity, muscle repair, and overall metabolic health. On these days, caloric intake is typically set at or above maintenance levels, which is the number of calories required to maintain current body weight without gaining or losing fat. For most individuals, this can range between 2000 to 2500 calories, but specific needs vary based on factors such as age, sex, weight, and activity level.

Purpose and Benefits:

1. **Prevent Metabolic Slowdown:** By periodically increasing caloric intake, high-calorie days help to prevent the body from entering a state of metabolic adaptation, where it slows down energy expenditure in response to prolonged calorie restriction.

2. **Muscle Preservation and Growth:** Adequate calorie intake supports muscle repair and growth, especially when paired with resistance training. This is crucial for endomorphs, who often struggle to maintain lean muscle mass while losing weight.

3. **Hormonal Balance:** Higher calorie consumption can positively impact hormones that regulate hunger and satiety, such as leptin and ghrelin. This helps in managing hunger levels and preventing binge eating.

Low-Calorie Days

Low-calorie days, in contrast, are designed to create a caloric deficit, prompting the body to utilize stored fat for energy. Caloric intake on these days is significantly reduced, typically ranging from 1200 to 1500 calories, depending on individual needs and goals.

Purpose and Benefits:

1. **Fat Loss:** The primary goal of low-calorie days is to induce a caloric deficit, leading to the breakdown of fat stores and weight loss. This is particularly beneficial for endomorphs, who have a higher tendency to store fat.
2. **Metabolic Flexibility:** Alternating between high and low-calorie days enhances the body's ability to efficiently switch between using carbohydrates and fats for energy, improving overall metabolic flexibility.
3. **Psychological Relief:** Knowing that high-calorie days are interspersed with low-calorie days can make the diet more psychologically sustainable, reducing feelings of deprivation and the likelihood of diet fatigue.

Implementation Strategies

To effectively implement high and low-calorie days, it is important to plan meals that are nutrient-dense and aligned with individual dietary preferences and goals. Here are some strategies:

1. **High-Calorie Days:**
    - Focus on balanced meals that include lean proteins, healthy fats, and complex carbohydrates.
    - Incorporate nutrient-dense foods such as whole grains, avocados, nuts, seeds, and lean meats.
    - Ensure adequate hydration and consider incorporating protein-rich snacks to support muscle repair.
2. **Low-Calorie Days:**
    - Prioritize high-protein foods and vegetables to maintain satiety while keeping calorie intake low.
    - Limit intake of high-calorie, low-nutrient foods such as processed snacks and sugary beverages.
    - Utilize meal planning and portion control to manage caloric intake effectively.

By understanding and implementing high-calorie and low-calorie days within a structured plan, individuals can maximize the benefits of calorie cycling, support metabolic health, and achieve sustainable weight loss. This balanced approach not only fosters a healthier relationship with food but also enhances long-term adherence to the diet, making it a viable strategy for endomorphs seeking effective weight management solutions.

Sample Calorie Cycling Schedules

Creating an effective calorie cycling schedule involves strategically alternating between high-calorie and low-calorie days to optimize metabolic function, enhance fat loss, and maintain muscle mass. Below are detailed examples of calorie cycling schedules tailored for different needs and lifestyles.

Example 1: Basic Alternating Schedule

Purpose: Ideal for beginners who want a straightforward approach to calorie cycling.

Schedule:

- **Monday:** High-calorie day (2000-2200 calories)
- **Tuesday:** Low-calorie day (1200-1400 calories)

- **Wednesday:** High-calorie day (2000-2200 calories)
- **Thursday:** Low-calorie day (1200-1400 calories)
- **Friday:** High-calorie day (2000-2200 calories)
- **Saturday:** Low-calorie day (1200-1400 calories)
- **Sunday:** High-calorie day (2000-2200 calories)

Rationale:

- **High-calorie days:** Provide necessary energy for intense workouts, support muscle repair, and prevent metabolic slowdown.
- **Low-calorie days:** Create a caloric deficit to promote fat loss while maintaining overall balance throughout the week.

Example 2: 5:2 Schedule

Purpose: Suitable for individuals who prefer a less frequent but more intense calorie cycling approach.

Schedule:

- **Monday to Friday:** Low-calorie days (1200-1400 calories each day)
- **Saturday:** High-calorie day (2500-2700 calories)
- **Sunday:** High-calorie day (2500-2700 calories)

Rationale:

- **Five consecutive low-calorie days:** Create a sustained caloric deficit, maximizing fat burning throughout the workweek.
- **Two consecutive high-calorie days:** Replenish glycogen stores, support recovery, and prevent adaptive thermogenesis.

Example 3: Fitness Enthusiast Schedule

Purpose: Designed for individuals who engage in regular high-intensity training sessions and need to align calorie intake with workout intensity.

Schedule:

- **Monday (Leg day):** High-calorie day (2500-2700 calories)
- **Tuesday (Rest day):** Low-calorie day (1200-1400 calories)
- **Wednesday (Upper body):** Moderate-calorie day (1800-2000 calories)
- **Thursday (Cardio):** Low-calorie day (1200-1400 calories)
- **Friday (Full body):** High-calorie day (2500-2700 calories)
- **Saturday (Active recovery):** Moderate-calorie day (1800-2000 calories)
- **Sunday (Rest day):** Low-calorie day (1200-1400 calories)

Rationale:

- **High-calorie days:** Coincide with intense workout sessions, ensuring adequate energy and nutrient availability for performance and recovery.

- **Low-calorie days:** Align with rest or light activity days, promoting fat loss without compromising muscle mass.
- **Moderate-calorie days:** Support active recovery and moderate workout sessions, providing balanced nutrition without overloading calories.

Example 4: Professional and Busy Lifestyle Schedule

Purpose: Tailored for individuals with demanding work schedules and limited time for meal planning.

Schedule:
- **Monday:** High-calorie day (2200-2400 calories)
- **Tuesday:** Low-calorie day (1200-1400 calories)
- **Wednesday:** Low-calorie day (1200-1400 calories)
- **Thursday:** High-calorie day (2200-2400 calories)
- **Friday:** Low-calorie day (1200-1400 calories)
- **Saturday:** High-calorie day (2200-2400 calories)
- **Sunday:** Low-calorie day (1200-1400 calories)

Rationale:
- **High-calorie days:** Placed strategically to allow flexibility for social events, family gatherings, or work functions.
- **Low-calorie days:** Interspersed to maintain a consistent caloric deficit, simplifying meal planning and adherence.

Tips for Implementing Calorie Cycling

1. **Monitor Progress:** Regularly track weight, body composition, and overall well-being to assess the effectiveness of the schedule.
2. **Adjust as Needed:** Modify calorie intake based on individual progress, energy levels, and specific goals.
3. **Nutrient Quality:** Prioritize nutrient-dense foods on both high and low-calorie days to ensure adequate intake of vitamins, minerals, and essential nutrients.
4. **Hydration:** Maintain proper hydration to support metabolic processes and overall health.
5. **Consistency:** Adhere to the schedule consistently while allowing flexibility for adjustments based on personal needs and lifestyle changes.

By following these sample calorie cycling schedules, individuals can tailor their dietary intake to support metabolic health, promote fat loss, and maintain muscle mass, achieving their weight management goals effectively.

Macronutrient Management

Understanding and managing macronutrients—proteins, carbohydrates, and fats—are crucial for optimizing the Metabolic Confusion Diet, particularly for women with an endomorph body type. Macronutrients play distinct and vital roles in the body, influencing metabolism, energy levels, and overall health. In this subchapter, we will delve into the importance of balancing these macronutrients to maximize the benefits of the diet and facilitate a smooth transition from an endomorph to a more ectomorphic body composition.

Proteins are essential for muscle repair and growth, supporting a higher metabolic rate, and ensuring satiety. By incorporating an adequate amount of protein into the diet, endomorph women can help preserve lean muscle mass, which is crucial for maintaining a healthy metabolism during periods of caloric cycling.

Carbohydrates, while often scrutinized, are necessary for providing the body with immediate energy, especially on high-calorie days or during intense workouts. The key is to focus on complex carbohydrates that provide sustained energy and help stabilize blood sugar levels. This approach can mitigate the insulin sensitivity issues often experienced by endomorphs.

Fats, though calorie-dense, are indispensable for hormone production, nutrient absorption, and overall cellular function. Healthy fats, such as those from avocados, nuts, and olive oil, can be strategically incorporated into the diet to support metabolic health and provide long-lasting satiety.

By understanding the unique roles and benefits of each macronutrient, endomorph women can tailor their dietary intake to support metabolic confusion, enhance fat loss, and promote overall well-being. This subchapter will provide detailed guidance on how to effectively balance proteins, carbohydrates, and fats within the framework of the Metabolic Confusion Diet, ensuring a comprehensive and sustainable approach to weight management.

Importance of Protein, Carbs, and Fats

Proteins

Proteins are fundamental macronutrients that play a critical role in maintaining and repairing body tissues, including muscles. For endomorphs, proteins are particularly significant due to their impact on muscle mass and metabolic rate. Higher protein intake can aid in muscle synthesis, which is essential for boosting the basal metabolic rate (BMR). This increase in muscle mass helps the body burn more calories at rest, facilitating weight loss and metabolic efficiency.

Proteins also have a high thermic effect, meaning the body uses more energy to digest proteins compared to fats and carbohydrates. This thermogenic property makes protein a valuable component in the Metabolic Confusion Diet, as it supports increased energy expenditure. Additionally, proteins promote satiety, reducing overall calorie intake by curbing hunger and decreasing the likelihood of overeating.

Carbohydrates

Carbohydrates are the body's primary source of energy, especially vital for brain function and physical activity. For endomorphs, managing carbohydrate intake is crucial due to their propensity for insulin resistance and fat storage. The key is to focus on complex carbohydrates, such as whole grains, legumes, and vegetables, which provide a steady release of glucose into the bloodstream. This steady release helps maintain stable blood sugar levels and prevents insulin spikes that can lead to fat storage.

On high-calorie days, incorporating adequate carbohydrates can fuel intense workouts and support recovery, making them an integral part of the calorie cycling strategy. Conversely, on low-calorie days, reducing carbohydrate intake can help manage insulin sensitivity and promote fat burning.

Fats

Dietary fats are essential for numerous bodily functions, including hormone production, nutrient absorption, and cellular health. For endomorphs, incorporating healthy fats is important to support these functions while promoting satiety and metabolic health. Healthy fats, such as those found in avocados, nuts, seeds, and olive oil, provide essential fatty acids that the body cannot synthesize on its own.

Fats are energy-dense, providing 9 calories per gram, compared to 4 calories per gram from proteins and carbohydrates. This density makes them a valuable source of sustained energy, particularly on low-calorie days when maintaining energy levels can be challenging. Moreover, fats play a crucial role in the absorption of fat-soluble vitamins (A, D, E, and K), which are vital for overall health and wellbeing.

Adjusting Macronutrient Ratios for Optimal Results

Understanding Macronutrient Ratios

Adjusting macronutrient ratios is a strategic approach to optimize the benefits of the Metabolic Confusion Diet for endomorph women. The goal is to tailor the intake of proteins, carbohydrates, and fats to enhance metabolic function, support muscle synthesis, and facilitate effective weight loss. This personalized adjustment can significantly impact how the body responds to different phases of calorie cycling.

Protein: The Building Block

For endomorphs, a higher protein intake is often beneficial due to its role in muscle maintenance and metabolism. A common recommendation is to consume 30-35% of total daily calories from protein. This high protein ratio supports muscle repair and growth, especially important on both high-calorie and low-calorie days. During high-calorie days, increased protein intake helps build muscle mass, which in turn raises the basal metabolic rate. On low-calorie days, maintaining a high protein intake helps preserve muscle mass and prevent the body from entering a catabolic state, where muscle tissue is broken down for energy.

Carbohydrates: Energy and Performance

Carbohydrates should be adjusted based on activity levels and metabolic needs. For endomorphs, it is generally advisable to consume 25-30% of total daily calories from carbohydrates on low-calorie days. This lower intake helps manage insulin sensitivity and encourages the body to utilize stored fat for energy. On high-calorie days, increasing carbohydrate intake to 40-45% of total daily calories can provide the necessary fuel for intense workouts and recovery. This strategic increase ensures that the body has ample glycogen stores to support physical performance and muscle recovery.

Fats: Sustained Energy and Health

Fats play a critical role in hormone production, cell health, and energy provision. For endomorphs, adjusting fat intake to 30-35% of total daily calories can be effective. Healthy fats, such as those from avocados, nuts, seeds, and olive oil, should be prioritized. On low-calorie days, maintaining a higher fat intake helps sustain energy levels and promotes satiety, making it easier to adhere to the reduced calorie intake. On high-calorie days, a slightly lower fat intake (around 25-30%) can balance the increased carbohydrate consumption, ensuring that overall caloric intake remains in check.

Periodization and Flexibility

Adjusting macronutrient ratios should be dynamic and flexible, reflecting changes in activity levels, weight loss progress, and individual metabolic responses. For instance, during periods of high physical activity or intense training, slightly increasing carbohydrate intake can enhance performance and recovery. Conversely, during less active periods, reducing carbohydrate intake and increasing protein and fat intake can help manage weight and maintain muscle mass.

Monitoring and Adjustments

Regular monitoring of progress is essential for optimizing macronutrient ratios. This includes tracking weight, body composition, energy levels, and overall well-being. Adjustments should be made based on these observations, with a focus on achieving a balance that supports metabolic health and weight loss goals. Consulting with a nutritionist or dietitian can provide personalized guidance, ensuring that macronutrient adjustments are tailored to individual needs and preferences.

Chapter 3: 7 Pillars to Transition from Endomorph to Ectomorph

In this chapter, we delve into the seven foundational principles essential for transforming an endomorphic body type into a more ectomorphic physique. This transition is not merely about aesthetics but involves a comprehensive approach that includes dietary adjustments, exercise regimens, and lifestyle changes. Each pillar represents a critical component of this holistic transformation, providing a structured pathway to achieve sustainable weight loss, increased metabolic efficiency, and improved overall health. By understanding and implementing these seven pillars, you can create a tailored plan that addresses the unique challenges faced by endomorphs, paving the way to a leaner and more balanced body type.

Pillar 1: Personalized Nutrition

Personalized nutrition forms the cornerstone of any successful body transformation, particularly when transitioning from an endomorphic to an ectomorphic physique. This approach involves tailoring your diet to meet your unique metabolic needs, genetic predispositions, and lifestyle factors. Unlike one-size-fits-all diets, personalized nutrition acknowledges that each individual's body responds differently to various types and amounts of food.

For endomorphs, who typically have a slower metabolism and a higher propensity to store fat, a personalized nutritional plan is crucial. This includes calculating the precise caloric intake required to create a sustainable energy deficit without triggering metabolic slowdowns. It also involves optimizing macronutrient ratios—adjusting protein, carbohydrates, and fats to enhance metabolic efficiency and support muscle retention while promoting fat loss.

Furthermore, personalized nutrition takes into account food preferences, intolerances, and potential allergies, ensuring that the diet is not only effective but also enjoyable and easy to adhere to. By integrating nutrient-dense foods that stabilize blood sugar levels and sustain energy, this approach helps mitigate the common challenges faced by endomorphs, such as cravings and energy dips.

Through the application of scientific principles and ongoing monitoring, personalized nutrition empowers individuals to make informed dietary choices that align with their specific health goals. This tailored strategy is pivotal in fostering long-term dietary adherence, optimizing metabolic function, and ultimately facilitating the transition towards a leaner, more ectomorphic body type.

Crafting Your Meal Plans

Crafting effective meal plans is a fundamental aspect of personalized nutrition, especially for those aiming to transition from an endomorphic to an ectomorphic body type. This process involves several critical steps that ensure your dietary intake is both nutritionally balanced and aligned with your metabolic and fitness goals. Here's a detailed guide on how to craft your meal plans:

Step 1: Assessing Your Basal Metabolic Rate (BMR) and Total Daily Energy Expenditure (TDEE)

Begin by calculating your Basal Metabolic Rate (BMR), which represents the number of calories your body requires at rest. You can use the Harris-Benedict equation or other reliable methods. Next, determine your Total Daily Energy Expenditure (TDEE) by factoring in your physical activity level. This step provides a foundation for understanding your caloric needs.

Step 2: Establishing Caloric Intake Goals

Based on your BMR and TDEE, establish a caloric intake goal that creates a moderate deficit to promote fat loss without compromising muscle mass. For endomorphs, it is essential to avoid drastic calorie reductions that can slow metabolism. Aim for a deficit of 500-750 calories per day to ensure sustainable weight loss.

Step 3: Determining Macronutrient Ratios

Macronutrient management is crucial. Typically, a balanced approach for endomorphs transitioning to an ectomorphic body type might include:

- **Protein**: 30-35% of total daily calories. High protein intake supports muscle maintenance and repair.
- **Carbohydrates**: 30-40% of total daily calories. Choose complex carbohydrates that provide sustained energy and stabilize blood sugar levels.
- **Fats**: 25-30% of total daily calories. Incorporate healthy fats that support metabolic health and hormone production.

Step 4: Selecting Nutrient-Dense Foods

Focus on incorporating nutrient-dense foods that provide essential vitamins and minerals while maintaining a caloric deficit. Prioritize lean proteins (such as chicken, turkey, fish, and legumes), whole grains (like quinoa, brown rice, and oats), and healthy fats (such as avocados, nuts, seeds, and olive oil). Include a variety of fruits and vegetables to ensure a broad spectrum of micronutrients.

Step 5: Planning Balanced Meals

Structure your meals to include a balance of protein, carbohydrates, and fats. For instance, a typical meal might consist of grilled chicken (protein), quinoa (carbohydrates), and a mixed green salad with olive oil (fats). Ensure each meal is satisfying and keeps you full longer by including fiber-rich foods and adequate protein.

Step 6: Meal Timing and Frequency

Consider the timing and frequency of your meals. Eating smaller, more frequent meals can help regulate blood sugar levels and prevent overeating. However, some may prefer three balanced meals a day. Choose a pattern that aligns with your lifestyle and helps you stay consistent.

Step 7: Monitoring and Adjusting

Regularly monitor your progress and adjust your meal plans as needed. Keep track of your weight, body composition, and energy levels. If you notice plateaus or unwanted changes, revisit your caloric intake and macronutrient ratios. Flexibility and adaptability are key to long-term success.

Step 8: Staying Hydrated

Hydration is often overlooked but vital. Ensure you drink plenty of water throughout the day to support metabolic processes and overall health. Aim for at least 8-10 glasses of water daily, adjusting based on your activity level and climate.

By following these detailed steps, you can craft personalized meal plans that support your transition from an endomorphic to an ectomorphic body type. This structured approach ensures that your dietary intake is both effective and sustainable, promoting optimal health and body composition changes.

Foods to Embrace and Avoid

Crafting a successful nutrition plan for transitioning from an endomorphic to an ectomorphic body type requires a keen understanding of which foods to incorporate into your diet and which to avoid. This knowledge ensures that your body receives the necessary nutrients to support fat loss, muscle gain, and overall health.

Foods to Embrace

1. **Lean Proteins**
   - **Chicken Breast**: High in protein and low in fat, perfect for muscle repair and growth.
   - **Turkey**: A lean protein source that is versatile and nutrient-dense.
   - **Fish**: Especially fatty fish like salmon, rich in omega-3 fatty acids that support metabolic health.
   - **Eggs**: A complete protein source that also provides essential vitamins and minerals.
   - **Legumes**: Beans, lentils, and chickpeas are excellent plant-based protein sources with additional fiber.

2. **Complex Carbohydrates**
   - **Quinoa**: A complete protein that also provides fiber and essential amino acids.
   - **Brown Rice**: A whole grain that provides sustained energy and supports digestive health.
   - **Oats**: High in fiber, oats help maintain stable blood sugar levels and keep you full longer.
   - **Sweet Potatoes**: Rich in vitamins A and C, and provide a steady energy source.

3. **Healthy Fats**
   - **Avocados**: High in monounsaturated fats, which support heart health and provide satiety.
   - **Nuts and Seeds**: Almonds, chia seeds, and flaxseeds offer healthy fats and fiber.
   - **Olive Oil**: A source of healthy fats that can be used in cooking and dressings.
   - **Fatty Fish**: Salmon and mackerel are excellent sources of omega-3 fatty acids.

4. **Fruits and Vegetables**
   - **Leafy Greens**: Spinach, kale, and Swiss chard are low in calories but high in vitamins and minerals.
   - **Berries**: Blueberries, strawberries, and raspberries are rich in antioxidants and fiber.
   - **Cruciferous Vegetables**: Broccoli, cauliflower, and Brussels sprouts support detoxification processes.
   - **Citrus Fruits**: Oranges, lemons, and grapefruits are high in vitamin C and support immune function.

5. **Whole Grains**
   - **Whole Wheat Bread**: Provides fiber and essential nutrients, aiding in digestion and sustained energy.
   - **Barley**: High in fiber, barley supports heart health and stable blood sugar levels.
   - **Buckwheat**: A gluten-free grain that is high in protein and fiber.

Foods to Avoid

1. **Refined Carbohydrates**
    - **White Bread**: Lacks fiber and essential nutrients, leading to rapid spikes in blood sugar.
    - **Pastries and Sweets**: High in sugar and unhealthy fats, contributing to weight gain and metabolic issues.
    - **White Pasta**: Processed and stripped of nutrients, leading to quick blood sugar increases.
    - **Sugary Cereals**: Often high in refined sugars and low in nutritional value.
2. **Processed Foods**
    - **Fast Food**: Typically high in unhealthy fats, sodium, and empty calories.
    - **Processed Meats**: Sausages, hot dogs, and deli meats contain unhealthy preservatives and fats.
    - **Snack Foods**: Chips, crackers, and other packaged snacks often contain trans fats and high sodium levels.
3. **Sugary Beverages**
    - **Soda**: High in sugar and empty calories, leading to weight gain and metabolic syndrome.
    - **Energy Drinks**: Often contain high levels of sugar and artificial ingredients.
    - **Sweetened Coffee Drinks**: Loaded with sugar and unhealthy fats, negating the potential benefits of coffee.
4. **High-Fat Dairy Products**
    - **Full-Fat Cheese**: High in saturated fats, which can contribute to cardiovascular issues.
    - **Cream and Butter**: High in calories and saturated fats, best used sparingly.
5. **Alcohol**
    - **Beer and Cocktails**: High in calories and sugar, leading to weight gain and impaired metabolic function.
    - **Wine**: Even though some wine has health benefits in moderation, it still contains calories that can add up quickly.

By carefully selecting foods that promote health and avoiding those that hinder your progress, you can create a balanced and effective nutrition plan. Emphasizing nutrient-dense foods supports your metabolic goals and helps in achieving a leaner, more defined body.

Pillar 2: Mindfulness and Stress Management

The second pillar in transitioning from an endomorph to an ectomorph body type is mindfulness and stress management. The connection between mental well-being and physical health is profound, particularly in the context of weight management and metabolic health. Chronic stress can significantly impede weight loss efforts by disrupting hormonal balance and increasing the production of cortisol, a stress hormone known to promote fat storage, especially in the abdominal area.

Mindfulness, the practice of being fully present and engaged in the moment, can play a crucial role in managing stress and promoting healthier lifestyle choices. It helps in cultivating a heightened awareness of the body's signals, including hunger and satiety cues, which can prevent overeating and promote better food choices. Techniques such as mindful eating encourage slower, more deliberate consumption of food, allowing for better digestion and increased satisfaction from meals.

Moreover, incorporating stress management strategies such as meditation, deep breathing exercises, yoga, and adequate sleep can lead to a more balanced and harmonious state of mind. These practices help lower cortisol levels, reduce anxiety, and enhance overall emotional resilience. By integrating mindfulness and effective stress management techniques into your daily routine, you can create a supportive mental environment that enhances your physical transformation efforts.

This chapter delves into the science behind stress and its impact on the body, explores various mindfulness practices, and provides practical strategies for integrating these techniques into your lifestyle. By prioritizing mental well-being, you lay a solid foundation for sustained weight loss and overall health improvement, making it easier to achieve and maintain your desired body type.

Impact of Stress on Weight Loss

Stress, a ubiquitous element in modern life, profoundly affects the body's physiological processes, particularly those related to weight management. Understanding the impact of stress on weight loss is critical for anyone striving to transition from an endomorph to an ectomorph body type.

Hormonal Influence

The primary mechanism through which stress impacts weight is hormonal. When the body experiences stress, it activates the hypothalamic-pituitary-adrenal (HPA) axis, leading to the release of cortisol, commonly referred to as the "stress hormone." Cortisol plays a pivotal role in various bodily functions, including metabolism and fat storage. Elevated cortisol levels, especially when sustained over long periods, can lead to increased appetite, cravings for high-calorie foods, and the accumulation of visceral fat, particularly around the abdomen. This fat is not only aesthetically undesirable but also associated with numerous health risks, including cardiovascular disease and diabetes.

Metabolic Disruption

Chronic stress disrupts metabolic processes. Cortisol can interfere with insulin sensitivity, leading to higher blood sugar levels and increased fat storage. This metabolic disruption can make it difficult for endomorphs, who already have a tendency to store fat easily, to lose weight. Additionally, stress can alter the balance of other hormones such as ghrelin and leptin, which regulate hunger and satiety. Increased ghrelin levels can enhance hunger, while decreased leptin levels can impair the feeling of fullness, leading to overeating.

Behavioral Responses

Stress often triggers behavioral responses that can further hinder weight loss efforts. Many individuals resort to emotional eating as a coping mechanism, consuming comfort foods that are typically high in sugar, fat, and calories. This pattern, known as stress eating, can sabotage dietary efforts and lead to weight gain. Additionally, stress can reduce the motivation to engage in physical activity, exacerbating weight management challenges.

Sleep Disruption

Stress is a well-known disruptor of sleep patterns, leading to poor sleep quality and duration. Inadequate sleep can further elevate cortisol levels and disrupt the balance of hunger-regulating hormones, creating a vicious cycle that hampers weight loss. Lack of sleep also decreases energy levels, making it harder to maintain an active lifestyle and adhere to exercise routines.

Psychological Factors

The psychological burden of chronic stress can lead to a sense of helplessness and decreased motivation, which are detrimental to sustained weight loss efforts. Mental fatigue and burnout can make it challenging to adhere to dietary plans and exercise regimens, undermining progress towards achieving an ectomorph body type.

Techniques for Stress Reduction and Mindfulness

Effective stress reduction and mindfulness techniques are essential components of a holistic approach to weight loss, particularly for individuals with an endomorph body type who are seeking to transition towards a leaner, ectomorph physique. These techniques can help manage the physiological and psychological impacts of stress, thereby supporting metabolic function and weight management. Here, we detail several scientifically-backed strategies for reducing stress and cultivating mindfulness.

1. Mindfulness Meditation

Mindfulness meditation involves focusing on the present moment without judgment. This practice has been shown to reduce cortisol levels, improve emotional regulation, and enhance overall well-being. By dedicating just 10-20 minutes a day to mindfulness meditation, individuals can experience significant reductions in stress and improvements in their ability to manage cravings and emotional eating. Guided meditations, apps like Headspace or Calm, and mindfulness classes can provide structure and support for beginners.

2. Deep Breathing Exercises

Deep breathing exercises, such as diaphragmatic breathing, can activate the parasympathetic nervous system, which counteracts the stress response. Techniques like the 4-7-8 breath, where you inhale for four seconds, hold for seven seconds, and exhale for eight seconds, can quickly reduce anxiety and promote a sense of calm. Regular practice of deep breathing can improve cardiovascular function and lower blood pressure, contributing to overall health.

3. Progressive Muscle Relaxation (PMR)

Progressive muscle relaxation involves tensing and then slowly relaxing different muscle groups in the body. This technique helps reduce physical tension and stress, enhances body awareness, and can improve sleep quality. PMR can be particularly beneficial when practiced before bedtime to alleviate insomnia and promote restorative sleep.

4. Yoga and Tai Chi

Yoga and Tai Chi are mind-body practices that combine physical postures, breathing exercises, and meditation. These practices not only enhance physical flexibility and strength but also reduce stress and anxiety. Regular participation in yoga or Tai Chi has been associated with lower levels of cortisol, reduced symptoms of depression, and improved overall mental health. Classes are widely available both in-person and online, making it accessible for individuals with varying levels of experience.

5. Physical Exercise

Regular physical exercise is a powerful stress reliever. Activities such as walking, running, swimming, or cycling increase the production of endorphins, the body's natural mood lifters. Exercise also reduces levels of the body's stress hormones, such as adrenaline and cortisol. For endomorphs, combining aerobic exercise with strength training can optimize metabolic function and support weight loss goals. Aim for at least 150 minutes of moderate-intensity exercise per week, as recommended by health authorities.

6. Journaling

Journaling is an effective way to process emotions and reduce stress. Writing about thoughts and feelings can provide clarity, reduce anxiety, and improve mood. Keeping a stress journal can help identify stressors and develop strategies to manage them. Reflective journaling, where you focus on positive experiences and gratitude, can also enhance mental well-being and resilience.

7. Social Support

Building a strong social support network is crucial for stress management. Engaging with friends, family, or support groups provides emotional comfort and practical advice. Sharing experiences and challenges can reduce feelings of isolation and stress. Participating in group activities or seeking support from a therapist or counselor can further enhance mental health and stress resilience.

Pillar 3: Hormonal Balance

Hormonal balance plays a crucial role in the regulation of body weight, metabolism, and overall health, particularly for individuals with an endomorph body type. Hormones such as insulin, cortisol, thyroid hormones, and sex hormones (estrogen and testosterone) significantly influence how the body stores and burns fat, as well as how it manages hunger and satiety. Achieving and maintaining hormonal balance can thus be a game-changer in the quest for weight loss and optimal health.

Endomorphs often face challenges related to insulin sensitivity and higher levels of cortisol due to stress, which can promote fat storage and make weight loss more difficult. Balancing these hormones requires a multifaceted approach that includes dietary adjustments, regular physical activity, stress management techniques, and possibly medical interventions under the guidance of healthcare professionals.

This sub chapter delves into the intricate workings of key hormones and their impact on metabolism and weight regulation. By understanding these hormonal influences, you can implement targeted strategies to support hormonal health. We will explore dietary choices that stabilize blood sugar levels, exercise regimens that enhance insulin sensitivity, and lifestyle changes that mitigate stress and reduce cortisol levels.

Additionally, we will discuss the importance of sleep and its profound impact on hormonal regulation, as well as the potential need for medical evaluations to identify and address any underlying hormonal imbalances. By adopting these evidence-based practices, you can optimize your hormonal environment, making it more conducive to weight loss and overall well-being.

Embark on this journey towards hormonal harmony with the knowledge and tools necessary to transform your body and health, guided by scientific principles and practical advice tailored to the unique needs of endomorph women.

Understanding Hormones and Their Role

Hormones are biochemical messengers that play a pivotal role in regulating numerous physiological processes, including metabolism, appetite, fat storage, and energy expenditure. For endomorphs, whose bodies are predisposed to store fat more readily, understanding and managing hormonal influences is critical for effective weight loss and health optimization.

Key Hormones Influencing Weight and Metabolism

1. **Insulin:** Insulin, produced by the pancreas, is essential for regulating blood sugar levels. It facilitates the uptake of glucose by cells for energy production or storage as glycogen in the liver and muscles. However, excessive insulin levels, often resulting from high carbohydrate intake, can lead to insulin resistance. This condition causes cells to respond poorly to insulin, leading to elevated blood glucose levels and increased fat storage, particularly around the abdomen. Endomorphs are more susceptible to insulin resistance, making blood sugar management crucial.

2. **Cortisol:** Cortisol is a stress hormone released by the adrenal glands. It helps the body respond to stress by mobilizing energy reserves. Chronic stress and persistently high cortisol levels can lead

to increased appetite and cravings for high-calorie foods, promoting fat accumulation, especially visceral fat. Elevated cortisol also impairs insulin sensitivity, compounding the challenges faced by endomorphs.

3. **Thyroid Hormones:** The thyroid gland produces hormones such as thyroxine (T4) and triiodothyronine (T3), which regulate metabolic rate. Hypothyroidism, or underactive thyroid, can slow metabolism, leading to weight gain and difficulty losing weight. Ensuring thyroid health is vital for maintaining an efficient metabolism.

4. **Sex Hormones:** Estrogen and testosterone significantly influence body composition. In women, estrogen helps regulate fat distribution, often leading to fat storage in the hips and thighs. However, imbalances, such as estrogen dominance, can promote weight gain and make weight loss more challenging. Testosterone, though present in lower levels in women, supports muscle mass maintenance and fat loss. A decline in testosterone levels can lead to increased fat mass and reduced muscle mass.

5. **Leptin and Ghrelin:** Leptin and ghrelin are hormones that regulate hunger and satiety. Leptin, produced by fat cells, signals the brain to reduce appetite when fat stores are sufficient. Endomorphs may experience leptin resistance, where the brain does not respond adequately to leptin signals, leading to overeating. Ghrelin, known as the "hunger hormone," stimulates appetite. High levels of ghrelin can increase hunger, making it harder to adhere to a calorie-controlled diet.

Strategies for Hormonal Balance

Balancing these hormones involves a comprehensive approach:

- **Dietary Adjustments:** Focus on low-glycemic index foods to manage insulin levels. Incorporate lean proteins, healthy fats, and fiber-rich vegetables to stabilize blood sugar and support satiety.
- **Stress Management:** Techniques such as mindfulness, meditation, and adequate sleep can help lower cortisol levels.
- **Regular Exercise:** Engage in both aerobic and resistance training to improve insulin sensitivity and support thyroid function.
- **Medical Evaluation:** Periodic check-ups with a healthcare provider can identify hormonal imbalances, guiding appropriate interventions such as medication or hormone therapy if necessary.

Understanding and managing the hormonal landscape is crucial for endomorphs to achieve their weight loss goals and improve overall health. This holistic approach addresses the root causes of weight gain, enabling sustainable and effective results.

Natural Ways to Balance Hormones

Balancing hormones naturally involves lifestyle changes and dietary modifications that support the endocrine system's optimal functioning. By understanding and implementing these strategies, individuals, especially endomorphs, can enhance their metabolic health and improve their overall well-being. Here are detailed approaches to achieving hormonal balance naturally:

Dietary Adjustments

1. **Nutrient-Dense Foods:** Consuming a diet rich in whole, unprocessed foods provides the body with essential nutrients that support hormonal health. Key foods include:
    - **Leafy Greens:** Spinach, kale, and broccoli are high in vitamins and minerals that support detoxification and hormone production.

- **Healthy Fats:** Avocado, nuts, seeds, and olive oil provide omega-3 and omega-6 fatty acids, crucial for hormone synthesis.
- **Lean Proteins:** Fish, chicken, beans, and legumes help maintain muscle mass and stabilize blood sugar levels, reducing insulin spikes.

2. **Fiber Intake:** Fiber aids in the elimination of excess hormones, particularly estrogen, by promoting regular bowel movements. Foods high in fiber include vegetables, fruits, whole grains, and legumes.
3. **Avoid Refined Carbohydrates and Sugars:** Limiting intake of refined sugars and carbohydrates helps maintain stable blood sugar levels, reducing the risk of insulin resistance. Opt for whole grains like quinoa, brown rice, and oats instead.
4. **Phytoestrogens:** Foods like flaxseeds, soybeans, and lentils contain plant-based estrogens that can help balance estrogen levels in the body. These are particularly beneficial for women experiencing estrogen dominance.

Lifestyle Changes

1. **Regular Exercise:** Physical activity is crucial for balancing hormones. It enhances insulin sensitivity, reduces cortisol levels, and promotes the release of endorphins, which improve mood. A combination of aerobic exercises, such as walking or swimming, and strength training exercises, like weight lifting, is recommended.
2. **Adequate Sleep:** Quality sleep is vital for hormonal balance. During sleep, the body regulates cortisol and growth hormone levels. Aim for 7-9 hours of sleep per night and maintain a consistent sleep schedule.
3. **Stress Management:** Chronic stress elevates cortisol levels, disrupting hormonal balance. Implement stress-reducing techniques such as:
   - **Mindfulness Meditation:** Practicing mindfulness can lower cortisol levels and improve overall emotional well-being.
   - **Yoga and Deep Breathing Exercises:** These activities promote relaxation and reduce stress hormone production.
4. **Hydration:** Drinking sufficient water supports the body's detoxification processes and ensures efficient hormone transport. Aim for at least 8 glasses of water per day.

Supplementation

1. **Adaptogenic Herbs:** Adaptogens like ashwagandha, rhodiola, and holy basil help the body adapt to stress and support adrenal gland function. These herbs can reduce cortisol levels and enhance resilience to stress.
2. **Vitamin and Mineral Supplements:**
   - **Vitamin D:** Essential for maintaining hormonal balance, vitamin D can be obtained through sunlight exposure and supplements.
   - **Magnesium:** Magnesium supports numerous biochemical reactions, including hormone synthesis. Foods high in magnesium include almonds, spinach, and dark chocolate, or consider a magnesium supplement.
3. **Probiotics:** Gut health is closely linked to hormone balance. Probiotic-rich foods like yogurt, kefir, sauerkraut, and supplements can support a healthy gut microbiome, aiding in hormone regulation.

Avoiding Endocrine Disruptors

1. **Reduce Exposure to Toxins:** Endocrine disruptors found in plastics, pesticides, and household chemicals can interfere with hormonal balance. To minimize exposure:
    - Use glass or stainless steel containers instead of plastic.
    - Choose organic produce to reduce pesticide intake.
    - Use natural cleaning products and personal care items.
2. **Avoid Excessive Caffeine and Alcohol:** High intake of caffeine and alcohol can disrupt hormonal balance by affecting the adrenal glands and liver. Limit caffeine to one cup of coffee per day and consume alcohol in moderation.

Implementing these natural strategies can significantly contribute to hormonal balance, improving metabolic health and overall well-being. By focusing on diet, lifestyle changes, supplementation, and reducing exposure to toxins, individuals can support their endocrine system and achieve their health goals more effectively.

Pillar 4: Fitness and Exercise

Fitness and exercise are critical components of achieving and maintaining a healthy body composition, particularly for individuals with an endomorph body type. Regular physical activity not only aids in weight loss but also enhances metabolic function, boosts energy levels, and improves overall physical and mental health. Understanding the unique needs of an endomorph body type can help tailor an effective exercise regimen that maximizes results.

Endomorphs typically have a higher percentage of body fat and a slower metabolism, making it more challenging to lose weight. However, a well-structured fitness program that combines both cardiovascular and resistance training can significantly improve metabolic rate and support the transition towards a leaner physique. Cardiovascular exercises, such as running, swimming, or cycling, are essential for burning calories and improving heart health. These activities help create a calorie deficit, which is crucial for weight loss.

Resistance training, on the other hand, is vital for building and maintaining muscle mass. Muscle tissue burns more calories at rest compared to fat tissue, thus increasing the resting metabolic rate. Incorporating weight lifting, bodyweight exercises, and resistance band workouts into the fitness routine can help endomorphs enhance their muscle mass and strength, leading to more efficient fat burning.

Moreover, incorporating flexibility and balance exercises, such as yoga or Pilates, can aid in muscle recovery and prevent injuries, ensuring a sustainable and long-term exercise regimen. These practices also promote mindfulness and stress reduction, which can positively impact hormonal balance and overall well-being.

The key to success lies in consistency and progression. By gradually increasing the intensity and variety of workouts, individuals can avoid plateaus and continue making progress. Understanding the importance of fitness and exercise in the context of an endomorph body type provides a comprehensive approach to achieving lasting health and fitness goals. This chapter will guide you through designing an effective and sustainable exercise plan tailored to your specific needs, ensuring you can embrace a healthier, more active lifestyle.

Best Exercises for Endomorphs

For individuals with an endomorph body type, the focus of an exercise regimen should be on activities that enhance metabolic rate, promote fat loss, and build muscle mass. Understanding the best types of exercises tailored to the physiological characteristics of endomorphs can lead to more effective and sustainable results. Below are the key categories of exercises that are most beneficial for endomorphs:

1. Cardiovascular Exercises

Cardiovascular exercises, or aerobic activities, are essential for burning calories and improving cardiovascular health. These exercises increase the heart rate and help create the necessary calorie deficit for weight loss. For endomorphs, high-intensity and moderate-intensity cardio sessions can be particularly effective.

- **High-Intensity Interval Training (HIIT):** HIIT involves short bursts of intense exercise followed by brief periods of rest or low-intensity exercise. This method is highly effective for burning calories and boosting metabolism. Examples include sprinting, cycling, or circuit training with minimal rest.
- **Steady-State Cardio:** Engaging in longer, consistent cardio sessions such as jogging, brisk walking, swimming, or cycling at a moderate intensity can also help burn a significant number of calories. Aim for at least 150 minutes of moderate-intensity aerobic activity per week.

2. Resistance Training

Building and maintaining muscle mass is crucial for endomorphs as muscle tissue increases the resting metabolic rate, aiding in continuous calorie burning even at rest. Incorporating resistance training into the fitness routine is essential for achieving this.

- **Weight Lifting:** Using free weights, machines, or resistance bands to perform exercises like squats, deadlifts, bench presses, and rows helps in building muscle strength and mass.
- **Bodyweight Exercises:** Push-ups, pull-ups, lunges, and planks are effective bodyweight exercises that can be performed anywhere and require no equipment. These exercises also improve functional strength and muscle tone.
- **Compound Movements:** Focus on compound movements that work multiple muscle groups simultaneously. Examples include squats with shoulder presses, deadlifts with rows, and lunges with bicep curls.

3. Flexibility and Balance Exercises

Flexibility and balance exercises support muscle recovery, reduce the risk of injury, and improve overall physical performance. These exercises also promote relaxation and mental well-being.

- **Yoga:** Practicing yoga enhances flexibility, balance, and muscular endurance. It also helps in stress reduction, which can positively influence hormonal balance and weight management.
- **Pilates:** Pilates focuses on core strength, stability, and flexibility. It is particularly beneficial for improving posture and overall body awareness.

4. Functional Training

Functional training involves exercises that mimic everyday movements, enhancing overall strength and coordination. This type of training is beneficial for improving performance in daily activities and preventing injuries.

- **Kettlebell Workouts:** Kettlebell swings, Turkish get-ups, and goblet squats are excellent for building functional strength and cardiovascular endurance.
- **Medicine Ball Exercises:** Medicine ball throws, slams, and rotational exercises engage the core and improve power and coordination.

Designing an Exercise Plan

To maximize the benefits of these exercises, it is crucial to design a balanced workout plan that incorporates a mix of cardiovascular, resistance, flexibility, and functional training. Here is a sample weekly exercise plan for endomorphs:

- **Monday:** HIIT session (30 minutes) + Flexibility exercises (15 minutes)
- **Tuesday:** Weight lifting (upper body focus)
- **Wednesday:** Steady-state cardio (45 minutes)
- **Thursday:** Weight lifting (lower body focus) + Core exercises
- **Friday:** Functional training (kettlebell or medicine ball workout)
- **Saturday:** Yoga or Pilates session (60 minutes)
- **Sunday:** Active recovery (light walking or stretching)

By consistently following a structured and varied exercise plan, endomorphs can enhance their metabolic efficiency, promote fat loss, and build lean muscle mass, leading to improved overall health and well-being.

Combining Cardio and Strength Training

Combining cardiovascular (cardio) exercises and strength training is a powerful strategy for endomorphs aiming to optimize fat loss, increase muscle mass, and improve overall fitness. This dual approach leverages the unique benefits of both exercise modalities, creating a synergistic effect that enhances metabolic function and promotes sustainable weight management. Below, we delve into the principles, benefits, and practical implementation of combining cardio and strength training.

Principles of Combining Cardio and Strength Training

1. **Sequential Training:** This approach involves performing cardio and strength training in the same workout session but in a sequential order. Typically, starting with strength training followed by cardio is recommended. Strength exercises deplete glycogen stores, allowing the body to shift to fat oxidation during subsequent cardio sessions.

2. **Concurrent Training:** In this method, cardio and strength exercises are alternated within the same workout session. For instance, a set of resistance exercises can be followed by a brief cardio interval, and this pattern is repeated. This approach is often used in circuit training and high-intensity interval training (HIIT).

3. **Periodized Training:** This strategy involves alternating focus between cardio and strength training on different days of the week. For example, strength training might be emphasized on certain days, while other days focus on cardio. This method allows for adequate recovery and adaptation.

Benefits of Combining Cardio and Strength Training

1. **Enhanced Fat Loss:** Cardio exercises increase calorie expenditure, while strength training builds muscle mass, which elevates resting metabolic rate. The combination accelerates fat loss by creating a significant caloric deficit and enhancing metabolic activity.

2. **Improved Cardiovascular Health:** Regular cardio exercise strengthens the heart and improves cardiovascular function, reducing the risk of heart disease. When combined with strength training, it ensures a balanced approach to heart health and muscular strength.

3. **Increased Muscle Mass and Strength:** Strength training promotes muscle hypertrophy and strength gains. By integrating cardio, you also enhance muscular endurance, allowing for better performance in both aerobic and anaerobic activities.

4. **Better Metabolic Flexibility**: Alternating between cardio and strength exercises enhances the body's ability to switch between using carbohydrates and fats as fuel. This metabolic flexibility is beneficial for overall energy management and weight control.
5. **Time Efficiency**: Combining both types of training in a single workout session maximizes time efficiency. This approach is ideal for individuals with busy schedules, ensuring they achieve comprehensive fitness benefits without needing to spend excessive time in the gym.

Practical Implementation of Combined Training

1. **Integrated Workouts**: Design workouts that include both cardio and strength elements. For example:
    - **Warm-up**: 5-10 minutes of light cardio (e.g., brisk walking, jogging).
    - **Strength Training**: 30 minutes focusing on major muscle groups (e.g., squats, deadlifts, bench press).
    - **Cardio Session**: 20-30 minutes of moderate-intensity cardio (e.g., cycling, elliptical).
    - **Cool-down**: 5-10 minutes of light stretching and mobility exercises.
2. **Circuit Training**: Create a circuit that alternates between strength and cardio exercises:
    - **Example Circuit**:
        - Squats (strength)
        - Jump rope (cardio)
        - Push-ups (strength)
        - High knees (cardio)
        - Rows (strength)
        - Burpees (cardio)
    - Perform each exercise for 1 minute, followed by a 15-second rest. Repeat the circuit 3-4 times.
3. **HIIT Workouts**: Incorporate HIIT sessions that blend short bursts of intense cardio with strength exercises:
    - **Example HIIT Session**:
        - 30 seconds sprint (cardio)
        - 30 seconds rest
        - 30 seconds kettlebell swings (strength)
        - 30 seconds rest
        - Repeat for 20-30 minutes.
4. **Periodized Schedule**: Alternate cardio and strength training on different days:
    - **Monday**: Strength training (upper body)
    - **Tuesday**: Cardio (steady-state or HIIT)

- **Wednesday**: Strength training (lower body)
- **Thursday**: Cardio (steady-state or HIIT)
- **Friday**: Full-body strength training
- **Saturday**: Cardio (steady-state or HIIT)
- **Sunday**: Active recovery (light stretching, yoga)

Monitoring and Adjusting Your Routine

1. **Progressive Overload**: Gradually increase the intensity, duration, and complexity of both cardio and strength exercises to continue making progress.
2. **Recovery**: Ensure adequate recovery between sessions to prevent overtraining and injury. Incorporate rest days and prioritize sleep and nutrition.
3. **Assessment**: Regularly assess your progress and make adjustments based on your goals and physical responses. Track metrics such as body composition, strength gains, and cardiovascular fitness improvements.

By thoughtfully combining cardio and strength training, endomorphs can achieve a balanced, effective, and sustainable fitness regimen that supports their weight loss and overall health goals.

Pillar 5: Sustainable Lifestyle Changes

Embarking on a journey to transition from an endomorph to an ectomorph body type requires more than just short-term dietary adjustments and exercise routines. Sustainable lifestyle changes are crucial for achieving long-term success and maintaining a healthier body composition. This chapter delves into the essential habits and practices that underpin a sustainable lifestyle, ensuring that the progress made through personalized nutrition, stress management, hormonal balance, and fitness routines is preserved and enhanced over time.

A sustainable approach to lifestyle changes involves integrating healthy habits into your daily routine in a way that feels natural and manageable. This means making gradual, consistent changes that you can stick with, rather than drastic alterations that are difficult to maintain. Key components of sustainable lifestyle changes include mindful eating, maintaining a balanced diet, regular physical activity, adequate sleep, and stress management. These elements work synergistically to support overall health and well-being.

Moreover, the chapter will emphasize the importance of setting realistic goals and celebrating small victories along the way. Recognizing and rewarding your progress fosters motivation and helps build a positive relationship with the changes you are making. Additionally, understanding the role of social support and community in maintaining a healthy lifestyle is critical. Engaging with like-minded individuals, whether through support groups, online communities, or fitness clubs, can provide encouragement, accountability, and shared experiences.

Incorporating these sustainable lifestyle changes into your daily life will not only aid in achieving your desired body type but also improve your overall quality of life. This chapter aims to equip you with the knowledge and strategies needed to create lasting, positive habits that support your health and fitness goals.

Building Healthy Habits

Building healthy habits is the cornerstone of achieving and maintaining a successful transition from an endomorph to an ectomorph body type. This subchapter provides a detailed exploration of how to establish and sustain beneficial behaviors that support your health and fitness goals.

Understanding Habits and Their Formation

Habits are automatic behaviors triggered by specific cues in our environment. They form through a process called habituation, where repeated actions become second nature over time. Understanding this process is critical in making lasting changes. The habit loop consists of three components: cue, routine, and reward. Identifying and manipulating these components can help create new, healthier habits.

Start Small and Be Consistent

One of the most effective strategies for building healthy habits is to start small. Implementing minor changes in your daily routine can lead to significant, long-term results. For example, instead of committing to an hour-long workout every day, begin with a 10-minute exercise routine and gradually increase the duration as it becomes part of your routine. Consistency is more important than intensity when establishing new habits.

Set Clear, Achievable Goals

Setting clear, specific, and achievable goals is essential for habit formation. Goals should be SMART: Specific, Measurable, Achievable, Relevant, and Time-bound. For instance, rather than setting a vague goal to "eat healthier," specify that you will "include a serving of vegetables in every meal." This clarity provides a roadmap for your actions and makes it easier to track progress.

Use Positive Reinforcement

Positive reinforcement can significantly enhance habit formation. Rewarding yourself for sticking to new habits can create a positive association with the behavior, making it more likely to stick. Rewards can be tangible, like treating yourself to a new book, or intangible, such as the satisfaction of feeling healthier and more energized.

Identify and Address Barriers

Recognizing potential obstacles and developing strategies to overcome them is crucial for building healthy habits. Common barriers include lack of time, motivation, or resources. Solutions might involve scheduling workouts at a convenient time, finding a workout buddy for accountability, or choosing cost-effective healthy foods. Anticipating challenges and planning accordingly can prevent setbacks.

Monitor Progress and Adjust as Needed

Regularly monitoring your progress helps to reinforce new habits and make necessary adjustments. Keep a journal or use an app to track your habits, noting what works and what doesn't. Reflect on your successes and challenges, and be flexible in modifying your approach to better suit your needs and circumstances.

Cultivate a Supportive Environment

Creating an environment that supports your new habits can enhance your success. This might include organizing your home to make healthy choices easier, such as keeping nutritious foods visible and accessible, and storing junk food out of sight. Surround yourself with supportive individuals who encourage your efforts and share similar health goals.

Practice Patience and Persistence

Building healthy habits is a gradual process that requires patience and persistence. It's normal to encounter setbacks along the way, but it's important to stay committed to your goals. Remember that forming new habits takes time, and each small step forward is a move towards a healthier, more sustainable lifestyle.

By implementing these strategies, you can effectively build and maintain healthy habits that support your journey from an endomorph to an ectomorph body type. These habits will not only facilitate your physical transformation but also enhance your overall well-being and quality of life.

Maintaining Consistency

Maintaining consistency is fundamental to achieving and sustaining your health and fitness goals, particularly when transitioning from an endomorph to an ectomorph body type. This subchapter delves into the strategies and principles necessary to maintain a consistent approach to diet, exercise, and overall lifestyle changes.

The Importance of Routine

Establishing a daily routine is crucial for maintaining consistency. Routines create a structured framework that makes it easier to incorporate healthy habits into your daily life. A well-planned routine ensures that diet, exercise, and self-care activities are prioritized, reducing the likelihood of neglecting these important aspects due to time constraints or other commitments.

Setting Realistic Expectations

Setting realistic expectations is essential for maintaining consistency. Unrealistic goals can lead to frustration and demotivation if they are not met. Instead, set achievable milestones that are challenging yet attainable. This approach fosters a sense of accomplishment and encourages continued adherence to your health plan.

Tracking Progress

Regularly tracking your progress is a powerful tool for maintaining consistency. Use journals, apps, or spreadsheets to log your daily activities, dietary intake, and exercise routines. Monitoring progress helps identify patterns, recognize achievements, and make necessary adjustments. It also serves as a motivational tool by visually demonstrating your improvements over time.

Building a Support Network

Having a support network can significantly enhance consistency. Engage family, friends, or join support groups that share similar health goals. A supportive environment provides encouragement, accountability, and motivation. Discuss your goals with your support network and seek their assistance in maintaining your commitment to your health plan.

Flexible Adaptation

Flexibility is key to maintaining consistency over the long term. Life events, work commitments, and unforeseen circumstances can disrupt your routine. Developing a flexible approach allows you to adapt your plan without abandoning your goals. For instance, if you miss a scheduled workout, find an alternative time to exercise or opt for a shorter, more intense session.

Prioritizing Self-Care

Self-care is an integral part of maintaining consistency. Adequate sleep, stress management, and mental health care are vital components of a healthy lifestyle. Ensure you allocate time for relaxation and activities that promote mental well-being. A balanced approach to self-care enhances overall health and supports sustained commitment to your fitness goals.

Leveraging Technology

Utilize technology to aid consistency in your health regimen. Fitness apps, meal planning tools, and wearable devices can provide reminders, track progress, and offer valuable insights into your habits. Technology can streamline your routine, making it easier to adhere to your dietary and exercise plans.

Staying Motivated

Maintaining motivation is critical for consistency. Identify intrinsic and extrinsic motivators that inspire you to stay committed. Intrinsic motivators include personal satisfaction, improved health, and the joy of achieving goals. Extrinsic motivators might involve rewards, social recognition, or achieving a desired physical appearance. Regularly revisit these motivators to reinforce your commitment.

Overcoming Plateaus

Plateaus are a common challenge in any health journey. When progress stalls, it can be discouraging. To overcome plateaus, vary your exercise routines, adjust dietary plans, and seek new challenges. Incorporating different activities and modifying intensity levels can stimulate progress and prevent stagnation.

Seeking Professional Guidance

Professional guidance from dietitians, nutritionists, and fitness trainers can provide personalized advice and support. Regular consultations ensure you are on the right track and help address any specific challenges you encounter. Expert input can refine your approach, making your efforts more effective and sustainable.

By implementing these strategies, you can maintain the consistency necessary to successfully transition from an endomorph to an ectomorph body type. Consistency is not about perfection but about persistent effort and dedication to your health and fitness goals.

Pillar 6: Community and Support

The journey towards achieving your health and fitness goals can be challenging, and the importance of a supportive community cannot be overstated. This chapter emphasizes the critical role that community and support play in the successful transition from an endomorph to an ectomorph body type. Leveraging the power of community provides a network of encouragement, accountability, and shared experiences that are invaluable for maintaining motivation and consistency.

A supportive community can take many forms, from friends and family to online forums and local fitness groups. Engaging with others who share similar goals creates a sense of belonging and mutual understanding, making the journey less isolating and more collaborative. The encouragement and positive reinforcement from peers can significantly boost morale, especially during challenging times or when progress seems slow.

Additionally, professional support from dietitians, fitness trainers, and healthcare providers is essential for personalized guidance and expert advice. These professionals offer tailored strategies and insights that can help you navigate obstacles and optimize your approach to diet and exercise. Regular consultations with experts ensure that your plan remains effective and aligned with your specific needs and goals.

Moreover, community support fosters a sense of accountability. Sharing your progress with others and setting collective goals can motivate you to stay committed. Knowing that others are invested in your success can provide the extra push needed to adhere to your regimen, even when motivation wanes.

Online communities and social media groups also offer a wealth of resources, from workout plans and nutritional advice to motivational stories and troubleshooting tips. These platforms allow for the exchange of knowledge and experiences, providing diverse perspectives and solutions to common challenges.

Importance of Social Support

Social support is a critical element in the successful implementation and maintenance of any health and fitness regimen, particularly when aiming to transition from an endomorph to an ectomorph body type. This section delves into the multifaceted importance of social support, underscoring its role in enhancing motivation, providing emotional reinforcement, and fostering a sense of accountability.

Enhancing Motivation

One of the primary benefits of social support is its ability to boost motivation. Engaging in a fitness journey can be daunting, and maintaining consistent motivation over time is challenging. Social support from friends, family, and fitness communities can provide the necessary encouragement to persevere through difficult periods. When motivation dips, a supportive network can reignite your drive by celebrating small victories and reminding you of your long-term goals. This reinforcement helps sustain the positive momentum required to achieve substantial body composition changes.

Providing Emotional Reinforcement

Emotional reinforcement from a social support network plays a crucial role in mitigating the psychological stresses associated with weight loss and body transformation efforts. The process of adopting new dietary habits and rigorous exercise routines can be emotionally taxing, often leading to feelings of frustration, anxiety, or self-doubt. Supportive interactions with others who understand or share similar experiences can offer comfort and empathy, alleviating these negative emotions. This emotional backing is vital for maintaining mental health and ensuring a positive mindset, which is essential for long-term success.

Fostering Accountability

Accountability is another significant aspect of social support. Sharing your goals and progress with a supportive community creates a sense of responsibility to adhere to your commitments. Knowing that others are aware of your journey and are invested in your success can provide a compelling incentive to stay on track. This accountability can be reinforced through regular check-ins, shared goal-setting, and participation in group activities or challenges. The collective nature of these activities fosters a disciplined approach to maintaining healthy habits and achieving milestones.

Encouraging Adherence to Healthy Behaviors

Social support also enhances adherence to prescribed health behaviors by providing practical assistance and shared resources. Friends or family members can participate in exercise routines, share healthy recipes, or offer logistical support, such as childcare or transportation, to facilitate your adherence to your fitness and nutrition plans. This practical support reduces barriers to healthy behaviors, making it easier to integrate them into daily life.

Building a Sense of Community

Finally, social support cultivates a sense of community and belonging, which is crucial for psychological well-being. Being part of a group with common goals fosters camaraderie and mutual respect. This sense of belonging can be a powerful motivator, as it provides an environment where members can share experiences, exchange advice, and celebrate successes together. The shared journey creates a bond that enhances the overall experience, making the pursuit of health and fitness more enjoyable and sustainable.

How to Build Your Support Network

Building a robust support network is an essential strategy for anyone undertaking significant lifestyle changes, particularly when aiming to transition from an endomorph to an ectomorph body type. A well-rounded support network can provide the motivation, accountability, and practical assistance necessary to sustain long-term health and fitness goals. This section provides a comprehensive guide on how to effectively build and maintain your support network.

Identifying Potential Supporters

The first step in building a support network is identifying individuals who can offer encouragement, advice, and companionship. These supporters can come from various areas of your life:

- **Family Members:** Close family members who understand your goals and challenges can offer daily emotional support and practical help.
- **Friends:** Friends who share similar health interests or have experience with fitness journeys can provide motivation and companionship during workouts.
- **Colleagues:** Workplace colleagues can become workout buddies or part of a lunch group focused on healthy eating.
- **Healthcare Professionals:** Nutritionists, personal trainers, and physicians can offer expert advice and personalized guidance.
- **Fitness Communities:** Joining local fitness groups, clubs, or online forums can connect you with like-minded individuals on similar journeys.

Engaging with Supportive Communities

Actively engaging with communities dedicated to health and fitness is crucial. These communities can be physical, such as local gym groups, or virtual, such as online fitness forums and social media groups. To engage effectively:

- **Join Fitness Classes:** Participating in group fitness classes or workshops can help you meet people with similar interests and goals.
- **Attend Health Seminars and Workshops:** These events provide valuable knowledge and opportunities to connect with professionals and peers.
- **Participate in Online Forums:** Websites and social media platforms offer numerous groups where you can share experiences, seek advice, and receive encouragement.

Communicating Your Goals

Clearly communicating your health and fitness goals to your support network ensures that everyone understands what you are striving to achieve and how they can help. This communication involves:

- **Sharing Your Vision:** Explain your long-term goals and the reasons behind your desire to transition body types.
- **Detailing Your Plan:** Outline the specific actions you plan to take, including your diet, exercise routines, and any professional help you are seeking.
- **Asking for Specific Support:** Whether it's a workout partner, someone to share healthy recipes with, or emotional support, be explicit about the kind of assistance you need.

Maintaining Regular Check-Ins

Regular check-ins with your support network help maintain accountability and provide opportunities to celebrate progress or address challenges. These check-ins can be:

- **Scheduled Meetings:** Set up regular meetings or calls with key supporters to discuss progress and setbacks.

- **Fitness Trackers:** Use apps or fitness trackers that allow you to share your activity and achievements with your network.
- **Social Media Updates:** Posting updates on social media can keep your broader network informed and engaged in your journey.

Leveraging Technology

Technology can enhance your support network by providing tools for communication, tracking progress, and accessing resources. Consider:

- **Fitness Apps:** Apps like MyFitnessPal, Strava, or Fitbit allow you to track your activity and share results with friends.
- **Virtual Workouts:** Participate in live or recorded workout sessions with instructors and peers through platforms like Zoom or Peloton.
- **Online Communities:** Engage with health and fitness communities on social media platforms like Facebook, Reddit, or Instagram.

Encouraging Reciprocal Support

A support network thrives on mutual encouragement and shared goals. Encourage reciprocal support by:

- **Supporting Others:** Offer encouragement, share advice, and celebrate the achievements of others in your network.
- **Creating Challenges:** Initiate group challenges or competitions to keep everyone motivated and engaged.
- **Sharing Resources:** Exchange information on nutrition, workouts, and wellness tips to benefit the entire network.

Evaluating and Adjusting Your Network

Periodically evaluate the effectiveness of your support network and make adjustments as needed. Consider:

- **Assessing Support Levels:** Identify which supporters are providing valuable assistance and which relationships might need strengthening or re-evaluation.
- **Expanding Your Network:** Continually seek out new members who can offer fresh perspectives and additional support.
- **Providing Feedback:** Offer constructive feedback to your supporters about how they can better assist you, and be open to receiving feedback in return.

Pillar 7: Tracking and Adjusting

Effective weight management and body transformation hinge on meticulous tracking and the willingness to make informed adjustments along the way. The process of transitioning from an endomorph to an ectomorph body type requires not just initial commitment but ongoing evaluation and fine-tuning. This pillar emphasizes the importance of consistent monitoring and the strategic adjustments necessary to optimize results.

Tracking involves systematically recording your dietary intake, exercise routines, and physiological changes. This data collection serves multiple purposes: it provides a clear picture of your progress, highlights areas that need improvement, and helps identify patterns that may be hindering your success.

Tools such as food diaries, fitness apps, and biometric measurements (like weight, body fat percentage, and muscle mass) are invaluable for maintaining an accurate record of your journey.

Adjusting, on the other hand, is about being responsive to the data you collect. It means interpreting the tracked information to make necessary changes in your nutrition plan, exercise regimen, and lifestyle habits. For example, if progress stalls, you might need to adjust macronutrient ratios, increase the intensity of workouts, or incorporate more rest and recovery into your routine. This dynamic approach ensures that your plan remains effective and tailored to your body's evolving needs.

By committing to diligent tracking and being proactive in making adjustments, you can overcome plateaus and continue progressing toward your goals. This process requires a blend of patience, persistence, and flexibility, acknowledging that the path to transformation is rarely linear but is navigable with the right tools and mindset.

Monitoring Progress

Monitoring progress is a critical aspect of any successful weight management and body transformation plan. It involves systematically tracking various metrics that provide insight into how your body responds to your dietary and exercise regimes. Effective monitoring allows you to stay informed about your progress, make timely adjustments, and maintain motivation throughout your journey.

Key Metrics to Track

1. **Body Weight**: Regularly weighing yourself provides a basic but useful measure of overall progress. It's important to weigh yourself under consistent conditions, such as at the same time of day and on the same day each week, to minimize variability.

2. **Body Measurements**: Using a tape measure to record measurements of key body areas (such as the waist, hips, thighs, and arms) can reveal changes in body composition that may not be reflected on the scale. These measurements can indicate fat loss and muscle gain.

3. **Body Fat Percentage**: Tracking your body fat percentage gives a more accurate picture of changes in body composition than weight alone. Methods such as skinfold calipers, bioelectrical impedance scales, or DEXA scans can be used for this purpose.

4. **Muscle Mass**: Monitoring changes in muscle mass is crucial, especially when aiming to transition from an endomorph to an ectomorph body type. Resistance training and protein intake should support muscle growth, and tools like bioelectrical impedance analysis (BIA) or DEXA scans can help track this.

5. **Dietary Intake**: Keeping a detailed food diary helps you monitor caloric intake and macronutrient distribution. Apps like MyFitnessPal or Cronometer can simplify this process by providing comprehensive databases and tracking features.

6. **Physical Performance**: Recording your performance in workouts, such as the weights lifted, repetitions completed, and cardio durations, helps track improvements in strength and endurance. Progressive increases in these metrics indicate positive adaptations to your exercise regimen.

7. **Biomarkers**: Periodic blood tests to monitor biomarkers such as cholesterol levels, blood glucose, and inflammatory markers can provide insight into how your diet and exercise program impact your overall health.

Tools for Monitoring

1. **Fitness Apps**: Applications like MyFitnessPal, FitBit, and Apple Health offer integrated solutions for tracking diet, exercise, and biometric data.

2. **Wearable Devices**: Fitness trackers and smartwatches can monitor daily activity levels, heart rate, and sleep patterns, offering a comprehensive view of your lifestyle habits.

3. **Journals and Logs**: Maintaining a physical or digital journal to log daily food intake, exercise routines, and subjective measures like energy levels and mood can provide a holistic view of your progress.

Interpreting Data

Understanding the data you collect is essential for making informed decisions. Look for trends over time rather than fixating on daily fluctuations, which can be influenced by numerous factors such as hydration status and meal timing. Regularly reviewing this data helps identify areas needing adjustment, ensuring your plan remains effective and aligned with your goals.

Monitoring progress is not only about tracking numbers but also about staying attuned to how you feel. Increased energy levels, improved sleep quality, and enhanced mood are significant indicators of progress that should not be overlooked.

By diligently monitoring these metrics and using them to guide your decisions, you can ensure that your journey toward transforming your body is both informed and effective.

Making Adjustments to Stay on Track

Making adjustments to your dietary and exercise regimen is crucial for maintaining momentum and achieving your long-term goals. The process involves evaluating the data you've collected, understanding what it indicates about your progress, and making informed changes to overcome plateaus or inefficiencies. Here's a detailed guide on how to make effective adjustments:

Assessing Your Data

1. **Review Progress Regularly**: Regular reviews of your progress data (weekly or bi-weekly) are essential. Look for trends in weight, body measurements, body fat percentage, muscle mass, and performance metrics.

2. **Identify Patterns**: Determine if there are consistent patterns or irregularities. For example, if weight loss has stalled or muscle gain is slower than expected, these trends need addressing.

3. **Consider External Factors**: Recognize external factors that may affect your progress, such as stress, sleep, illness, or lifestyle changes. These can significantly impact your body's response to diet and exercise.

Adjusting Your Diet

1. **Caloric Intake**: If weight loss has plateaued, consider a slight reduction in daily caloric intake. Ensure the reduction is moderate (around 100-200 calories) to avoid triggering metabolic adaptation and excessive hunger.

2. **Macronutrient Ratios**: Re-evaluate your macronutrient distribution. For example, increasing protein intake can support muscle maintenance and satiety, while adjusting carbohydrate and fat intake can optimize energy levels and fat loss.

3. **Meal Timing**: Adjust the timing of your meals and snacks to better support your energy needs and metabolic rate. Consider incorporating nutrient-dense, lower-calorie foods to enhance satiety and nutrient intake without excess calories.

4. **Hydration and Supplements**: Ensure adequate hydration and consider dietary supplements if necessary, such as omega-3 fatty acids, vitamin D, or a multivitamin to fill nutritional gaps.

Adjusting Your Exercise Regimen

1. **Intensity and Volume**: If your progress in muscle gain or strength has slowed, consider increasing the intensity or volume of your workouts. This might involve lifting heavier weights, increasing the number of sets or repetitions, or incorporating more challenging exercises.

2. **Variety in Exercises**: Incorporate new exercises to target different muscle groups and prevent adaptation. This can include variations of your current exercises or entirely new movements that challenge your body in different ways.

3. **Cardiovascular Exercise**: Evaluate the amount and type of cardio you're doing. If fat loss has stalled, consider adding high-intensity interval training (HIIT) sessions, which can boost calorie burn and improve cardiovascular fitness without requiring excessive time.

4. **Rest and Recovery**: Ensure you're getting adequate rest between workouts. Overtraining can lead to plateaus and injuries. Incorporate rest days and focus on recovery strategies such as stretching, foam rolling, and adequate sleep.

Behavioral and Lifestyle Adjustments

1. **Stress Management**: Address any increases in stress that may be affecting your progress. Techniques such as mindfulness, meditation, or engaging in relaxing activities can help mitigate stress-related barriers to progress.

2. **Sleep Quality**: Ensure you are getting sufficient and quality sleep, as inadequate sleep can impair recovery, hormone balance, and overall progress. Aim for 7-9 hours of sleep per night.

3. **Consistency and Accountability**: Stay consistent with your efforts and hold yourself accountable. Consider working with a coach or joining a support group to maintain motivation and adherence to your plan.

Reevaluating Goals

1. **Set Realistic Milestones**: Reassess your short-term and long-term goals to ensure they remain realistic and achievable based on your progress. Adjust them as needed to keep yourself motivated and focused.

2. **Celebrate Small Wins**: Recognize and celebrate small achievements along the way. This can boost morale and help maintain a positive outlook on your journey.

By systematically reviewing your progress and making thoughtful adjustments, you can overcome obstacles and continue moving toward your goals effectively. The key is to remain flexible and responsive to your body's feedback, ensuring that your plan evolves with your progress.

Chapter 4: Recipes for Success

Low-Calorie Breakfast Recipes

Avocado and Egg White Scramble

Preparation Time: 5 minutes
Cooking Time: 5 minutes
Servings: 1
Ingredients:
- 3 large egg whites
- 1/2 ripe avocado, diced
- 1 small tomato, diced
- 1 tablespoon olive oil
- Salt and pepper to taste

Procedure:
1. **Heat the Pan:** In a non-stick skillet, heat the olive oil over medium heat.
2. **Cook the Egg Whites:** Pour the egg whites into the skillet. Cook, stirring frequently, until they are fully set but still soft, about 2-3 minutes.
3. **Add Vegetables:** Gently fold in the diced avocado and tomato. Cook for an additional 1-2 minutes, just until the avocado is warm.
4. **Season and Serve:** Season with salt and pepper to taste. Serve immediately.

Macronutrients (per serving):
- **Calories:** 220 kcal
- **Carbohydrates:** 6g
- **Fat:** 16g
- **Protein:** 12g

Berry Protein Smoothie

Preparation Time: 5 minutes
Cooking Time: 0 minutes
Servings: 1
Ingredients:
- 1 cup mixed berries (strawberries, blueberries, raspberries)
- 1 scoop vanilla protein powder
- 1/2 cup unsweetened almond milk
- 1/2 cup plain Greek yogurt
- 1 tablespoon chia seeds

Procedure:
1. **Combine Ingredients:** Place the mixed berries, vanilla protein powder, unsweetened almond milk, plain Greek yogurt, and chia seeds in a blender.
2. **Blend:** Blend on high until the mixture is smooth and creamy.
3. **Adjust Consistency:** If the smoothie is too thick, add a little more almond milk and blend again until you reach your desired consistency.
4. **Serve:** Pour the smoothie into a glass and enjoy immediately.

Macronutrients (per serving):
- **Calories:** 260 kcal
- **Carbohydrates:** 28g
- **Fat:** 5g
- **Protein:** 27g

Chia Seed Pudding with Almond Milk

Preparation Time: 5 minutes
Cooking Time: 0 minutes
Servings: 1
Ingredients:
- 3 tablespoons chia seeds
- 1 cup unsweetened almond milk
- 1 teaspoon vanilla extract
- 1 teaspoon honey or maple syrup (optional, for sweetness)
- Fresh berries or sliced almonds for topping (optional)

Procedure:
1. **Combine Ingredients:** In a bowl or mason jar, mix the chia seeds, unsweetened almond milk, and vanilla extract. Add honey or maple syrup if using for sweetness.
2. **Stir Well:** Stir the mixture thoroughly to ensure the chia seeds are evenly distributed and not clumped together.
3. **Refrigerate:** Cover the bowl or jar and refrigerate for at least 2 hours, or overnight, to allow the chia seeds to absorb the liquid and thicken into a pudding-like consistency.
4. **Serve:** Before serving, give the pudding a good stir. Top with fresh berries or sliced almonds if desired, and enjoy!

Macronutrients (per serving):
- **Calories:** 200 kcal
- **Carbohydrates:** 18g
- **Fat:** 11g
- **Protein:** 6g

Cottage Cheese and Berry Bowl

Preparation Time: 5 minutes
Cooking Time: 0 minutes
Servings: 1
Ingredients:
- 1 cup low-fat cottage cheese
- 1/2 cup mixed fresh berries (strawberries, blueberries, raspberries)
- 1 tablespoon honey or maple syrup (optional, for sweetness)
- 1 tablespoon chia seeds or flax seeds (optional, for added texture and nutrients)
- A few fresh mint leaves for garnish (optional)

Procedure:
1. **Assemble Ingredients:** Place the low-fat cottage cheese in a serving bowl.
2. **Add Berries:** Top the cottage cheese with mixed fresh berries.
3. **Add Sweetener:** Drizzle honey or maple syrup over the berries and cottage cheese if using.
4. **Garnish and Serve:** Sprinkle chia seeds or flax seeds on top for added texture and nutrients. Garnish with fresh mint leaves if desired. Serve immediately and enjoy!

Macronutrients (per serving):
- **Calories:** 220 kcal
- **Carbohydrates:** 20g
- **Fat:** 5g
- **Protein:** 25g

Greek Yogurt with Flaxseeds and Blueberries

Preparation Time: 5 minutes
Cooking Time: 0 minutes
Servings: 1
Ingredients:
- 1 cup Greek yogurt (plain, non-fat)
- 1/2 cup fresh blueberries
- 1 tablespoon ground flaxseeds
- 1 teaspoon honey (optional, for sweetness)
- A pinch of cinnamon (optional, for flavor)

Procedure:
1. **Prepare the Yogurt:** Place the Greek yogurt in a serving bowl.
2. **Add Blueberries:** Top the yogurt with fresh blueberries.
3. **Sprinkle Flaxseeds:** Sprinkle ground flaxseeds over the yogurt and blueberries.
4. **Add Sweetener and Flavor:** Drizzle honey over the mixture if desired for sweetness and add a pinch of cinnamon for extra flavor. Mix gently and serve immediately.

Macronutrients (per serving):
- **Calories:** 210 kcal
- **Carbohydrates:** 22g
- **Fat:** 5g
- **Protein:** 20g

Kale and Spinach Smoothie

Preparation Time: 5 minutes
Cooking Time: 0 minutes
Servings: 1
Ingredients:
- 1 cup kale leaves (stems removed)
- 1 cup spinach leaves
- 1 medium banana
- 1 cup unsweetened almond milk
- 1 tablespoon chia seeds

Procedure:
1. **Prepare Ingredients:** Rinse the kale and spinach leaves thoroughly.
2. **Blend Base:** Add the kale, spinach, and almond milk to a blender. Blend until smooth.
3. **Add Banana and Chia Seeds:** Add the banana and chia seeds to the blender. Blend again until fully combined and smooth.
4. **Serve:** Pour the smoothie into a glass and enjoy immediately.

Macronutrients (per serving):
- **Calories:** 210 kcal
- **Carbohydrates:** 32g
- **Fat:** 6g
- **Protein:** 6g

Quinoa Breakfast Bowl with Vegetables

Preparation Time: 10 minutes
Cooking Time: 15 minutes
Servings: 2
Ingredients:
- 1 cup cooked quinoa
- 1/2 cup cherry tomatoes, halved
- 1/2 cup spinach leaves
- 1/4 cup chopped bell peppers
- 1 tablespoon olive oil

Procedure:
1. **Cook Quinoa:** If not already cooked, prepare quinoa according to package instructions.
2. **Sauté Vegetables:** In a medium skillet, heat olive oil over medium heat. Add cherry tomatoes, spinach, and bell peppers. Sauté for 3-5 minutes until vegetables are tender.
3. **Combine Ingredients:** In a bowl, combine the cooked quinoa and sautéed vegetables. Mix well.
4. **Serve:** Divide the mixture into two bowls and serve immediately.

Macronutrients (per serving):
- **Calories:** 280 kcal
- **Carbohydrates:** 34g
- **Fat:** 12g
- **Protein:** 8g

Quinoa Breakfast Bowl with Vegetables

Preparation Time: 10 minutes
Cooking Time: 15 minutes
Servings: 1
Ingredients:
- 1/2 cup cooked quinoa
- 1/4 cup cherry tomatoes, halved
- 1/4 cup spinach leaves
- 1/4 cup chopped bell peppers
- 1 teaspoon olive oil

Procedure:
1. **Cook Quinoa:** If not already cooked, prepare quinoa according to package instructions.
2. **Sauté Vegetables:** In a small skillet, heat olive oil over medium heat. Add cherry tomatoes, spinach, and bell peppers. Sauté for 3-5 minutes until vegetables are tender.
3. **Combine Ingredients:** In a bowl, combine the cooked quinoa and sautéed vegetables. Mix well.
4. **Serve:** Transfer the mixture into a serving bowl and serve immediately.

Macronutrients (per serving):
- **Calories:** 210 kcal
- **Carbohydrates:** 26g
- **Fat:** 9g
- **Protein:** 6g

Scrambled Tofu with Spinach and Tomatoes

Preparation Time: 10 minutes
Cooking Time: 10 minutes
Servings: 1
Ingredients:
- 1/2 cup firm tofu, crumbled
- 1/2 cup spinach leaves
- 1/4 cup cherry tomatoes, halved
- 1 teaspoon olive oil
- 1/4 teaspoon turmeric (optional for color)

Procedure:
1. **Prepare Tofu:** Crumble the firm tofu into small pieces with your hands or a fork.
2. **Cook Tofu:** In a small skillet, heat olive oil over medium heat. Add the crumbled tofu and turmeric (if using). Cook for 3-4 minutes, stirring occasionally.
3. **Add Vegetables:** Add the spinach leaves and cherry tomatoes to the skillet. Cook for an additional 3-4 minutes until the spinach is wilted and the tomatoes are soft.
4. **Serve:** Transfer the scrambled tofu with spinach and tomatoes to a plate and serve immediately.

Macronutrients (per serving):
- **Calories:** 180 kcal
- **Carbohydrates:** 8g
- **Fat:** 12g
- **Protein:** 12g

Zucchini and Carrot Pancakes

Preparation Time: 10 minutes
Cooking Time: 10 minutes
Servings: 1
Ingredients:
- 1/2 cup grated zucchini
- 1/2 cup grated carrot
- 1 large egg
- 2 tablespoons whole wheat flour
- 1 teaspoon olive oil

Procedure:
1. **Prepare Vegetables:** Grate the zucchini and carrot, then place them in a bowl. Press with a paper towel to remove excess moisture.
2. **Mix Ingredients:** In a mixing bowl, combine the grated zucchini, grated carrot, egg, and whole wheat flour. Mix until well combined.
3. **Cook Pancakes:** Heat olive oil in a non-stick skillet over medium heat. Scoop spoonfuls of the mixture onto the skillet, flattening each scoop to form pancakes. Cook for 3-4 minutes on each side until golden brown.
4. **Serve:** Transfer the pancakes to a plate and serve warm.

Macronutrients (per serving):
- **Calories:** 180 kcal
- **Carbohydrates:** 14g
- **Fat:** 10g
- **Protein:** 8g

Low-Calorie Lunch Recipes

Baked Cod with Asparagus

Preparation Time: 10 minutes
Cooking Time: 20 minutes
Servings: 1 person
Ingredients
- 1 cod fillet (about 150g)
- 1 cup asparagus spears, trimmed
- 1 tablespoon olive oil
- 1 clove garlic, minced
- Salt and pepper to taste

Procedure
1. **Preheat Oven:** Preheat the oven to 375°F (190°C). Line a baking sheet with parchment paper.
2. **Prepare Ingredients:** Place the cod fillet and asparagus spears on the baking sheet. Drizzle with olive oil and sprinkle with minced garlic, salt, and pepper.
3. **Bake:** Bake in the preheated oven for 20 minutes, or until the cod flakes easily with a fork and the asparagus is tender.
4. **Serve:** Remove from the oven and serve immediately. Enjoy your delicious and nutritious meal!

Macronutrients (per serving)
- **Calories:** 270 kcal
- **Carbohydrates:** 5g
- **Fat:** 14g
- **Protein:** 30g

Chicken and Avocado Salad

Preparation Time: 10 minutes
Cooking Time: 15 minutes
Servings: 1 person
Ingredients
- 1 cooked chicken breast (about 150g), shredded or chopped
- 1/2 avocado, diced
- 2 cups mixed greens (spinach, arugula, and lettuce)
- 1 tablespoon olive oil
- 1 tablespoon lemon juice

Procedure
1. **Prepare Ingredients:** In a large bowl, combine the shredded or chopped chicken breast, diced avocado, and mixed greens.
2. **Dress Salad:** In a small bowl, whisk together the olive oil and lemon juice. Season with salt and pepper to taste.
3. **Combine:** Drizzle the dressing over the salad and toss gently to combine all ingredients.
4. **Serve:** Transfer the salad to a serving plate and enjoy your fresh and nutritious meal.

Macronutrients (per serving)
- **Calories:** 350 kcal
- **Carbohydrates:** 10g
- **Fat:** 25g
- **Protein:** 30g

Chickpea and Spinach Stew

Preparation Time: 10 minutes
Cooking Time: 20 minutes
Servings: 1 person
Ingredients
- 1 cup canned chickpeas, drained and rinsed
- 2 cups fresh spinach
- 1/2 cup diced tomatoes (canned or fresh)
- 1 tablespoon olive oil
- 1 clove garlic, minced

Procedure
1. **Sauté Garlic:** Heat olive oil in a medium saucepan over medium heat. Add the minced garlic and sauté until fragrant, about 1 minute.
2. **Add Tomatoes and Chickpeas:** Add the diced tomatoes and chickpeas to the pan. Cook for 5 minutes, stirring occasionally.
3. **Add Spinach:** Add the fresh spinach to the pan and cook until wilted, about 3-5 minutes. Stir to combine all ingredients.
4. **Simmer:** Reduce heat to low and let the stew simmer for an additional 10 minutes, allowing the flavors to meld. Season with salt and pepper to taste.

Macronutrients (per serving)
- **Calories:** 280 kcal
- **Carbohydrates:** 35g
- **Fat:** 10g
- **Protein:** 10g

Grilled Salmon with Quinoa

Preparation Time: 10 minutes
Cooking Time: 20 minutes
Servings: 1 person
Ingredients
- 1 salmon fillet (about 4 oz)
- 1/2 cup quinoa
- 1 cup water
- 1 tablespoon olive oil
- Juice of 1/2 lemon

Procedure
1. **Cook Quinoa:** Rinse the quinoa under cold water. In a small pot, bring 1 cup of water to a boil. Add the quinoa, reduce heat to low, cover, and simmer for 15 minutes or until the water is absorbed and the quinoa is tender. Fluff with a fork.
2. **Prepare Salmon:** Preheat a grill or grill pan over medium-high heat. Brush the salmon fillet with olive oil and season with salt and pepper. Grill the salmon for about 4-5 minutes on each side, or until it flakes easily with a fork.
3. **Combine Ingredients:** Plate the cooked quinoa and top with the grilled salmon.
4. **Finish and Serve:** Squeeze the lemon juice over the salmon and quinoa for added flavor. Serve immediately.

Macronutrients (per serving)
- **Calories:** 430 kcal
- **Carbohydrates:** 36g
- **Fat:** 18g
- **Protein:** 33g

Lentil and Vegetable Soup

Preparation Time: 10 minutes
Cooking Time: 30 minutes
Servings: 1 person
Ingredients
- 1/4 cup dried lentils
- 1 small carrot, diced
- 1 small zucchini, diced
- 1 cup vegetable broth
- 1 tablespoon olive oil

Procedure
1. **Prepare Ingredients:** Rinse the lentils under cold water. Dice the carrot and zucchini into small pieces.
2. **Cook Lentils:** In a medium pot, heat the olive oil over medium heat. Add the diced carrot and zucchini, and sauté for about 5 minutes until they begin to soften.
3. **Simmer Soup:** Add the rinsed lentils and vegetable broth to the pot. Bring to a boil, then reduce the heat to low, cover, and simmer for 25-30 minutes, or until the lentils are tender.
4. **Serve:** Season with salt and pepper to taste. Serve hot.

Macronutrients (per serving)
- **Calories:** 280 kcal
- **Carbohydrates:** 36g
- **Fat:** 10g
- **Protein:** 10g

Shrimp and Zucchini Noodles

Preparation Time: 10 minutes
Cooking Time: 10 minutes
Servings: 1 person
Ingredients
- 1 medium zucchini, spiralized into noodles
- 100g shrimp, peeled and deveined
- 1 clove garlic, minced
- 1 tablespoon olive oil
- 1/4 teaspoon red pepper flakes (optional)

Procedure
1. **Prepare Ingredients:** Spiralize the zucchini into noodles using a spiralizer. Mince the garlic.
2. **Cook Shrimp:** In a large skillet, heat the olive oil over medium heat. Add the garlic and red pepper flakes (if using) and sauté for 1 minute. Add the shrimp and cook for 2-3 minutes on each side, until pink and opaque.
3. **Add Zucchini Noodles:** Add the zucchini noodles to the skillet and toss with the shrimp and garlic. Cook for 2-3 minutes until the zucchini noodles are slightly tender but still firm.
4. **Serve:** Season with salt and pepper to taste. Serve immediately.

Macronutrients (per serving)
- **Calories:** 220 kcal
- **Carbohydrates:** 8g
- **Fat:** 12g
- **Protein:** 20g

Spinach and Feta Stuffed Peppers

Preparation Time: 10 minutes
Cooking Time: 20 minutes
Servings: 1 person
Ingredients
- 1 large bell pepper, halved and seeds removed
- 1 cup fresh spinach, chopped
- 1/4 cup feta cheese, crumbled
- 1 small onion, finely chopped
- 1 tablespoon olive oil

Procedure
1. **Prepare Ingredients:** Preheat the oven to 375°F (190°C). Halve the bell pepper and remove seeds. Chop the spinach and onion finely.
2. **Sauté Filling:** In a skillet, heat the olive oil over medium heat. Add the chopped onion and sauté until translucent, about 3-4 minutes. Add the chopped spinach and cook until wilted, about 2 minutes. Remove from heat and stir in the crumbled feta cheese.
3. **Stuff Peppers:** Place the bell pepper halves on a baking sheet. Fill each half with the spinach and feta mixture.
4. **Bake and Serve:** Bake in the preheated oven for 15-20 minutes, until the peppers are tender and the filling is heated through. Serve immediately.

Macronutrients (per serving)
- **Calories:** 210 kcal
- **Carbohydrates:** 10g
- **Fat:** 15g
- **Protein:** 7g

Tofu and Broccoli Stir-Fry

Preparation Time: 10 minutes
Cooking Time: 10 minutes
Servings: 1 person
Ingredients
- 1/2 cup firm tofu, cubed
- 1 cup broccoli florets
- 1 tablespoon soy sauce (low sodium)
- 1 tablespoon olive oil
- 1 garlic clove, minced

Procedure
1. **Prepare Ingredients:** Cube the tofu and chop the broccoli into small florets. Mince the garlic.
2. **Cook Tofu:** In a large skillet or wok, heat the olive oil over medium-high heat. Add the cubed tofu and cook until golden brown on all sides, about 5-7 minutes. Remove tofu from the skillet and set aside.
3. **Sauté Broccoli:** In the same skillet, add the minced garlic and sauté for 1 minute. Add the broccoli florets and stir-fry for about 3-4 minutes until tender-crisp.
4. **Combine and Serve:** Return the tofu to the skillet with the broccoli. Pour in the soy sauce and stir well to combine. Cook for another 1-2 minutes to heat through. Serve immediately.

Macronutrients (per serving)
- **Calories:** 200 kcal
- **Carbohydrates:** 10g
- **Fat:** 14g
- **Protein:** 10g

Turkey Lettuce Wraps

Preparation Time: 10 minutes
Cooking Time: 10 minutes
Servings: 1 person
Ingredients
- 4 large lettuce leaves
- 1/2 cup ground turkey
- 1/4 cup diced bell pepper
- 1 tablespoon soy sauce (low sodium)
- 1 tablespoon olive oil

Procedure
1. **Prepare Ingredients:** Wash the lettuce leaves and pat them dry. Dice the bell pepper.
2. **Cook Turkey:** In a medium skillet, heat the olive oil over medium-high heat. Add the ground turkey and cook until browned, about 5-7 minutes. Break up the turkey into small pieces as it cooks.
3. **Add Vegetables:** Add the diced bell pepper to the skillet and cook for another 2-3 minutes until the pepper is tender. Stir in the soy sauce and cook for an additional minute to combine the flavors.
4. **Assemble Wraps:** Spoon the turkey and pepper mixture evenly onto the lettuce leaves. Wrap the lettuce around the filling to create wraps. Serve immediately.

Macronutrients (per serving)
- **Calories:** 220 kcal
- **Carbohydrates:** 4g
- **Fat:** 14g
- **Protein:** 18g

Zucchini and Tomato Salad

Preparation Time: 10 minutes
Cooking Time: 0 minutes
Servings: 1 person
Ingredients
- 1 small zucchini, thinly sliced
- 1 medium tomato, diced
- 1 tablespoon olive oil
- 1 tablespoon balsamic vinegar
- 1/4 teaspoon salt

Procedure
1. **Prepare Vegetables:** Wash the zucchini and tomato. Thinly slice the zucchini and dice the tomato.
2. **Combine Ingredients:** In a medium bowl, combine the sliced zucchini and diced tomato.
3. **Dress the Salad:** Drizzle the olive oil and balsamic vinegar over the vegetables. Sprinkle with salt.
4. **Toss and Serve:** Gently toss the salad to coat the vegetables evenly with the dressing. Serve immediately.

Macronutrients (per serving)
- **Calories:** 120 kcal
- **Carbohydrates:** 6g
- **Fat:** 10g
- **Protein:** 1g

Low-Calorie Dinner Recipes

Baked Lemon Herb Chicken

Preparation Time: 10 minutes
Cooking Time: 25 minutes
Servings: 1
Ingredients
- 1 chicken breast (about 6 oz)
- 1 tablespoon olive oil
- 1 tablespoon lemon juice
- 1 teaspoon mixed dried herbs (such as thyme, rosemary, and oregano)
- Salt and pepper to taste

Procedure
1. **Preheat Oven**: Preheat your oven to 400°F (200°C). Line a baking dish with parchment paper or lightly grease it.
2. **Prepare Chicken**: Place the chicken breast in the baking dish. Drizzle with olive oil and lemon juice. Sprinkle with mixed dried herbs, salt, and pepper.
3. **Bake**: Bake the chicken in the preheated oven for 25 minutes, or until the internal temperature reaches 165°F (74°C) and the chicken is cooked through.
4. **Serve**: Remove from the oven and let it rest for a few minutes before slicing. Serve with your favorite side of vegetables or salad.

Macronutrients
- **Calories**: 250 kcal
- **Carbohydrates**: 1g
- **Fat**: 14g
- **Protein**: 28g

Cauliflower Rice Stir-Fry

Preparation Time: 10 minutes
Cooking Time: 10 minutes
Servings: 1
Ingredients
- 1 cup cauliflower rice
- 1/2 cup mixed vegetables (e.g., bell peppers, carrots, peas)
- 1 tablespoon olive oil
- 1 tablespoon soy sauce (low sodium)
- 1 egg

Procedure
1. **Prepare Ingredients**: Heat the olive oil in a large skillet or wok over medium-high heat.
2. **Cook Vegetables**: Add the mixed vegetables to the skillet and stir-fry for about 5 minutes, or until they start to soften.
3. **Add Cauliflower Rice**: Add the cauliflower rice to the skillet and stir well. Pour the soy sauce over the mixture and stir-fry for another 3-4 minutes.
4. **Cook Egg**: Push the cauliflower rice and vegetables to one side of the skillet. Crack the egg into the empty side and scramble it. Once the egg is cooked, mix it into the cauliflower rice and vegetables. Cook for another minute until everything is well combined and heated through.

Macronutrients
- **Calories**: 180 kcal
- **Carbohydrates**: 10g
- **Fat**: 10g
- **Protein**: 8g

Garlic Butter Shrimp with Asparagus

Preparation Time: 10 minutes
Cooking Time: 10 minutes
Servings: 1
Ingredients
- 6 oz shrimp, peeled and deveined
- 1 cup asparagus, trimmed and cut into 2-inch pieces
- 1 tablespoon butter
- 2 cloves garlic, minced
- Salt and pepper to taste

Procedure
1. **Prepare Ingredients**: Heat the butter in a large skillet over medium heat until melted. Add the minced garlic and cook for about 1 minute, until fragrant.
2. **Cook Shrimp**: Add the shrimp to the skillet, season with salt and pepper, and cook for 2-3 minutes on each side until they turn pink and are cooked through. Remove the shrimp from the skillet and set aside.
3. **Cook Asparagus**: In the same skillet, add the asparagus pieces. Cook for about 5 minutes, stirring occasionally, until they are tender-crisp.
4. **Combine and Serve**: Return the shrimp to the skillet and mix with the asparagus until everything is well combined and heated through. Serve immediately.

Macronutrients
- **Calories**: 220 kcal
- **Carbohydrates**: 6g
- **Fat**: 10g
- **Protein**: 28g

Grilled Eggplant with Tahini Sauce

Preparation Time: 10 minutes
Cooking Time: 15 minutes
Servings: 1
Ingredients
- 1 medium eggplant, sliced into 1/2-inch rounds
- 1 tablespoon olive oil
- 2 tablespoons tahini
- 1 tablespoon lemon juice
- Salt and pepper to taste

Procedure
1. **Prepare Eggplant**: Preheat the grill to medium-high heat. Brush both sides of the eggplant slices with olive oil and season with salt and pepper.
2. **Grill Eggplant**: Place the eggplant slices on the grill. Cook for about 5-7 minutes on each side, until they are tender and have grill marks.
3. **Make Tahini Sauce**: In a small bowl, whisk together the tahini and lemon juice. If the sauce is too thick, add a small amount of water to reach the desired consistency. Season with salt to taste.
4. **Serve**: Arrange the grilled eggplant slices on a plate and drizzle with the tahini sauce. Serve immediately.

Macronutrients
- **Calories**: 210 kcal
- **Carbohydrates**: 15g
- **Fat**: 15g
- **Protein**: 4g

Herb-Crusted Tilapia

Preparation Time: 10 minutes
Cooking Time: 15 minutes
Servings: 1
Ingredients
- 1 tilapia fillet
- 1 tablespoon olive oil
- 1/4 cup whole wheat breadcrumbs
- 1 teaspoon dried mixed herbs (such as parsley, thyme, and oregano)
- Salt and pepper to taste

Procedure
1. **Prepare the Coating:** Preheat the oven to 375°F (190°C). In a small bowl, mix the whole wheat breadcrumbs with the dried mixed herbs, salt, and pepper.
2. **Coat the Tilapia:** Brush the tilapia fillet with olive oil, then press it into the breadcrumb mixture, ensuring it is well-coated on both sides.
3. **Bake the Tilapia:** Place the coated tilapia fillet on a baking sheet lined with parchment paper. Bake in the preheated oven for about 15 minutes, or until the fish is cooked through and the crust is golden brown.
4. **Serve:** Remove from the oven and let it rest for a couple of minutes. Serve hot with a side of steamed vegetables or a light salad.

Macronutrients
- **Calories:** 260 kcal
- **Carbohydrates:** 15g
- **Fat:** 12g
- **Protein:** 25g

Quinoa Stuffed Bell Peppers

Preparation Time: 15 minutes
Cooking Time: 25 minutes
Servings: 1
Ingredients
- 1 large bell pepper
- 1/2 cup cooked quinoa
- 1/4 cup black beans, drained and rinsed
- 1/4 cup diced tomatoes
- 1 tablespoon shredded low-fat cheese (optional)

Procedure
1. **Prepare the Bell Pepper:** Preheat the oven to 375°F (190°C). Cut the top off the bell pepper and remove the seeds and membranes. Set aside.
2. **Mix the Filling:** In a bowl, combine the cooked quinoa, black beans, and diced tomatoes. Mix well.
3. **Stuff the Pepper:** Spoon the quinoa mixture into the hollowed-out bell pepper. If using, sprinkle the shredded cheese on top.
4. **Bake:** Place the stuffed bell pepper in a baking dish and cover with foil. Bake for 20 minutes, then remove the foil and bake for an additional 5 minutes until the pepper is tender and the cheese is melted (if used). Serve hot.

Macronutrients
- **Calories:** 250 kcal
- **Carbohydrates:** 45g
- **Fat:** 4g
- **Protein:** 10g

Sprouts and Chicken

Preparation Time: 10 minutes
Cooking Time: 25 minutes
Servings: 1
Ingredients
- 1 boneless, skinless chicken breast (about 4 oz)
- 1 cup Brussels sprouts, halved
- 1 tablespoon olive oil
- 1/2 teaspoon garlic powder
- Salt and pepper to taste

Procedure
1. **Preheat Oven**: Preheat the oven to 400°F (200°C).
2. **Prepare Ingredients**: In a bowl, toss the Brussels sprouts with olive oil, garlic powder, salt, and pepper. Place the chicken breast on a baking sheet and season both sides with salt and pepper.
3. **Roast**: Arrange the Brussels sprouts around the chicken on the baking sheet. Roast in the preheated oven for 20-25 minutes, until the chicken is cooked through (internal temperature of 165°F or 74°C) and the Brussels sprouts are tender and slightly caramelized.
4. **Serve**: Remove from the oven and let the chicken rest for a few minutes before slicing. Serve the chicken slices with the roasted Brussels sprouts.

Macronutrients
- **Calories**: 320 kcal
- **Carbohydrates**: 12g
- **Fat**: 14g
- **Protein**: 38g

Salmon and Avocado Salad

Preparation Time: 10 minutes
Cooking Time: 10 minutes
Servings: 1
Ingredients
- 4 oz salmon fillet
- 1/2 avocado, sliced
- 2 cups mixed salad greens
- 1 tablespoon olive oil
- 1 tablespoon lemon juice
- Salt and pepper to taste

Procedure
1. **Cook the Salmon**: Season the salmon fillet with salt and pepper. Heat a non-stick skillet over medium heat and add the salmon. Cook for about 4-5 minutes on each side, or until the salmon is cooked through and flakes easily with a fork.
2. **Prepare the Dressing**: In a small bowl, whisk together the olive oil and lemon juice. Season with a pinch of salt and pepper.
3. **Assemble the Salad**: Arrange the mixed salad greens on a plate. Top with the sliced avocado and cooked salmon fillet.
4. **Dress and Serve**: Drizzle the lemon olive oil dressing over the salad. Serve immediately and enjoy.

Macronutrients
- **Calories**: 450 kcal
- **Carbohydrates**: 8g
- **Fat**: 34g
- **Protein**: 28g

Spaghetti Squash with Marinara Sauce

Preparation Time: 10 minutes
Cooking Time: 40 minutes
Servings: 1
Ingredients
- 1 small spaghetti squash
- 1 cup marinara sauce (preferably low-sodium)
- 1 tablespoon olive oil
- 1 clove garlic, minced
- 1 tablespoon grated Parmesan cheese (optional)
- Salt and pepper to taste

Procedure
1. **Prepare the Spaghetti Squash:** Preheat your oven to 400°F (200°C). Cut the spaghetti squash in half lengthwise and scoop out the seeds. Drizzle the insides with olive oil and season with salt and pepper. Place the squash halves cut-side down on a baking sheet and roast for 30-40 minutes, or until the flesh is tender and can be easily shredded with a fork.
2. **Cook the Marinara Sauce:** While the squash is roasting, heat a small saucepan over medium heat. Add a bit of olive oil and the minced garlic. Sauté until fragrant, about 1-2 minutes. Add the marinara sauce and let it simmer on low heat until the squash is ready.
3. **Shred the Squash:** Once the squash is cooked, use a fork to scrape out the flesh into spaghetti-like strands. Place the strands into a serving bowl.
4. **Assemble and Serve:** Pour the marinara sauce over the spaghetti squash strands and mix well. Top with grated Parmesan cheese, if desired. Serve immediately and enjoy!

Macronutrients
- **Calories:** 220 kcal
- **Carbohydrates:** 25g
- **Fat:** 12g
- **Protein:** 3g

Low-Calorie Snacks and Desserts Recipes

Apple Slices with Almond Butter

Preparation Time: 5 minutes
Cooking Time: None
Servings: 1
Ingredients:
- 1 medium apple (such as Fuji or Granny Smith)
- 2 tablespoons almond butter
- 1 teaspoon cinnamon (optional)
- 1 teaspoon chia seeds (optional)

Procedure:
1. **Wash and Slice Apple:** Wash the apple thoroughly. Slice the apple into thin wedges, removing the core.
2. **Prepare Almond Butter:** Place 2 tablespoons of almond butter in a small bowl. If desired, mix in 1 teaspoon of cinnamon for added flavor.
3. **Serve:** Arrange the apple slices on a plate. Drizzle or spread the almond butter over the apple slices.
4. **Optional Topping:** Sprinkle chia seeds over the top for an extra nutritional boost.

Macronutrients (Approximate):
- **Calories:** 220 kcal
- **Carbohydrates:** 26g
- **Fat:** 14g
- **Protein:** 4g

Berry Chia Pudding

Preparation Time: 5 minutes
Cooking Time: 0 minutes (requires refrigeration time: 4 hours or overnight)
Servings: 1
Ingredients:
- 1/2 cup unsweetened almond milk
- 2 tablespoons chia seeds
- 1/2 cup mixed berries (such as strawberries, blueberries, raspberries)
- 1 teaspoon honey or maple syrup (optional)
- 1/4 teaspoon vanilla extract (optional)

Procedure:
1. **Mix Ingredients:** In a bowl or a mason jar, combine the almond milk, chia seeds, honey or maple syrup, and vanilla extract. Stir well to ensure the chia seeds are evenly distributed.
2. **Refrigerate:** Cover the bowl or jar and refrigerate for at least 4 hours or overnight. Stir the mixture once or twice during the first hour to prevent the chia seeds from clumping together.
3. **Add Berries:** After the chia pudding has thickened, remove it from the refrigerator. Top with mixed berries.
4. **Serve:** Enjoy immediately, or store in the refrigerator for up to 2 days.

Macronutrients (Approximate):
- **Calories:** 180 kcal
- **Carbohydrates:** 25g
- **Fat:** 7g
- **Protein:** 4g

Cucumber and Hummus Bites

Preparation Time: 10 minutes
Cooking Time: 0 minutes
Servings: 1
Ingredients:
- 1/2 cucumber, sliced into rounds
- 2 tablespoons hummus
- 1 cherry tomato, quartered
- 1 teaspoon olive oil (optional)
- A pinch of paprika or black pepper for garnish

Procedure:
1. **Prepare Cucumber:** Wash the cucumber thoroughly and slice it into rounds about 1/4 inch thick.
2. **Add Hummus:** Spread a small dollop of hummus on each cucumber slice, about 1/2 teaspoon per slice.
3. **Top with Tomato:** Place a quarter of a cherry tomato on top of the hummus on each cucumber slice.
4. **Garnish:** Drizzle with a small amount of olive oil if desired and sprinkle with paprika or black pepper for an extra flavor boost.

Macronutrients (Approximate):
- **Calories:** 100 kcal
- **Carbohydrates:** 10g
- **Fat:** 5g
- **Protein:** 2g

Dark Chocolate Dipped Strawberries

Preparation Time: 10 minutes
Cooking Time: 5 minutes
Servings: 1
Ingredients:
- 6 fresh strawberries
- 2 ounces dark chocolate (70% cocoa or higher)
- 1 teaspoon coconut oil (optional for smoother chocolate)
- A pinch of sea salt (optional for garnish)
- A few chopped nuts or shredded coconut (optional for garnish)

Procedure:
1. **Prepare Strawberries:** Wash the strawberries and pat them dry with a paper towel. Make sure they are completely dry to ensure the chocolate adheres well.
2. **Melt Chocolate:** In a microwave-safe bowl, combine the dark chocolate and coconut oil (if using). Microwave in 20-second intervals, stirring after each, until the chocolate is completely melted and smooth.
3. **Dip Strawberries:** Hold each strawberry by the stem and dip it into the melted chocolate, covering about two-thirds of the berry. Allow any excess chocolate to drip off before placing the strawberry on a parchment-lined plate.
4. **Garnish and Set:** Sprinkle a pinch of sea salt, chopped nuts, or shredded coconut over the chocolate-coated strawberries if desired. Let them set at room temperature or refrigerate for a few minutes until the chocolate hardens.

Macronutrients (Approximate):
- **Calories:** 150 kcal
- **Carbohydrates:** 20g
- **Fat:** 8g
- **Protein:** 2g

Frozen Yogurt Blueberry Bites

Preparation Time: 10 minutes
Cooking Time: 0 minutes (plus freezing time)
Servings: 1
Ingredients:
- 1/2 cup fresh blueberries
- 1/2 cup Greek yogurt (plain or vanilla)
- 1 teaspoon honey or maple syrup (optional)
- 1/2 teaspoon vanilla extract (optional)
- 1 tablespoon granola (optional for topping)

Procedure:
1. **Prepare Yogurt Mixture:** In a small bowl, mix the Greek yogurt with honey or maple syrup and vanilla extract if using. Stir until well combined.
2. **Dip Blueberries:** Using a toothpick or small fork, dip each blueberry into the yogurt mixture, ensuring it is fully coated. Place the coated blueberries on a parchment-lined baking sheet or plate.
3. **Freeze:** Once all blueberries are coated and placed on the sheet, sprinkle granola over them if desired. Place the sheet in the freezer for at least 1 hour, or until the yogurt is completely frozen.
4. **Serve:** Once frozen, transfer the yogurt-covered blueberries to a small bowl or a resealable plastic bag for storage. Enjoy them straight from the freezer for a refreshing snack.

Macronutrients (Approximate):
- **Calories:** 120 kcal
- **Carbohydrates:** 20g
- **Fat:** 1g
- **Protein:** 7g

Greek Yogurt with Honey and Walnuts

Preparation Time: 5 minutes
Cooking Time: 0 minutes
Servings: 1
Ingredients:
- 1 cup Greek yogurt (plain)
- 1 tablespoon honey
- 2 tablespoons chopped walnuts
- 1/4 teaspoon cinnamon (optional)
- Fresh fruit for garnish (optional)

Procedure:
1. **Prepare Yogurt Base:** Place the Greek yogurt in a serving bowl.
2. **Add Honey:** Drizzle the honey evenly over the yogurt.
3. **Top with Walnuts:** Sprinkle the chopped walnuts on top of the yogurt and honey.
4. **Optional Garnishes:** Add a sprinkle of cinnamon for extra flavor and garnish with fresh fruit if desired.

Macronutrients (Approximate):
- **Calories:** 250 kcal
- **Carbohydrates:** 24g
- **Fat:** 12g
- **Protein:** 16g

Kale Chips

Preparation Time: 5 minutes
Cooking Time: 15 minutes
Servings: 1
Ingredients:
- 2 cups kale leaves, washed and dried
- 1 tablespoon olive oil
- 1/4 teaspoon salt
- 1/4 teaspoon garlic powder (optional)
- 1/4 teaspoon paprika (optional)

Procedure:
1. **Preheat Oven:** Preheat your oven to 350°F (175°C).
2. **Prepare Kale:** Remove the kale leaves from their stems and tear them into bite-sized pieces. Place the kale in a large bowl.
3. **Season Kale:** Drizzle the olive oil over the kale and sprinkle with salt. Add garlic powder and paprika if desired. Toss the kale until evenly coated.
4. **Bake Kale:** Spread the kale pieces in a single layer on a baking sheet. Bake for 10-15 minutes, or until the edges are brown but not burnt. Remove from the oven and let cool slightly before enjoying.

Macronutrients (Approximate):
- **Calories:** 120 kcal
- **Carbohydrates:** 7g
- **Fat:** 10g
- **Protein:** 3g

Protein-Packed Energy Balls

Preparation Time: 10 minutes
Cooking Time: None (chill time: 30 minutes)
Servings: 1 (makes about 4 energy balls)
Ingredients:
- 1/4 cup rolled oats
- 2 tablespoons natural peanut butter
- 1 tablespoon honey
- 1 tablespoon protein powder (vanilla or chocolate)
- 1 tablespoon mini dark chocolate chips (optional)

Procedure:
1. **Mix Ingredients:** In a medium bowl, combine the rolled oats, natural peanut butter, honey, protein powder, and mini dark chocolate chips (if using). Mix until well combined.
2. **Form Balls:** Using your hands, form the mixture into small balls (about 1-inch in diameter).
3. **Chill:** Place the energy balls on a plate or baking sheet and refrigerate for at least 30 minutes to firm up.
4. **Enjoy:** Once chilled, enjoy your protein-packed energy balls as a quick and healthy snack.

Macronutrients (Approximate per serving):
- **Calories:** 250 kcal
- **Carbohydrates:** 25g
- **Fat:** 12g
- **Protein:** 10g

Spiced Roasted Chickpeas

Preparation Time: 5 minutes
Cooking Time: 30 minutes
Servings: 1
Ingredients:
- 1/2 cup canned chickpeas, drained and rinsed
- 1 teaspoon olive oil
- 1/2 teaspoon paprika
- 1/4 teaspoon garlic powder
- 1/4 teaspoon sea salt

Procedure:
1. **Preheat Oven:** Preheat your oven to 400°F (200°C).
2. **Prepare Chickpeas:** Spread the drained and rinsed chickpeas on a paper towel and pat them dry. Remove any loose skins.
3. **Season Chickpeas:** In a bowl, toss the chickpeas with olive oil, paprika, garlic powder, and sea salt until evenly coated.
4. **Roast Chickpeas:** Spread the seasoned chickpeas in a single layer on a baking sheet. Roast in the preheated oven for 30 minutes, shaking the pan halfway through, until the chickpeas are crispy. Let cool slightly before enjoying.

Macronutrients (Approximate per serving):
- **Calories:** 180 kcal
- **Carbohydrates:** 24g
- **Fat:** 7g
- **Protein:** 7g

Zucchini Muffins

Preparation Time: 10 minutes
Cooking Time: 20 minutes
Servings: 1 (makes 2 muffins)
Ingredients:
- 1/2 cup grated zucchini
- 1 egg
- 1/4 cup almond flour
- 1 tablespoon honey
- 1/4 teaspoon baking powder

Procedure:
1. **Preheat Oven:** Preheat your oven to 350°F (175°C). Line a muffin tin with two paper liners or grease two muffin cups.
2. **Mix Ingredients:** In a bowl, whisk the egg and honey until well combined. Add the grated zucchini, almond flour, and baking powder. Mix until all ingredients are well incorporated.
3. **Fill Muffin Cups:** Divide the batter evenly between the two prepared muffin cups.
4. **Bake Muffins:** Bake in the preheated oven for 20 minutes, or until a toothpick inserted into the center of the muffins comes out clean. Let the muffins cool in the tin for a few minutes before transferring them to a wire rack to cool completely.

Macronutrients (Approximate per serving):
- **Calories:** 180 kcal
- **Carbohydrates:** 12g
- **Fat:** 10g
- **Protein:** 6g

High-Calorie Breakfast Recipes

Avocado Toast with Poached Egg

Preparation Time: 5 minutes
Cooking Time: 10 minutes
Servings: 1 person
Ingredients:
- 1 slice of whole grain bread
- 1/2 ripe avocado
- 1 large egg
- 1 teaspoon lemon juice
- Salt and pepper to taste

Procedure:
1. **Toast the Bread:**
   - Toast the slice of whole grain bread until golden and crispy.
2. **Prepare the Avocado:**
   - In a small bowl, mash the avocado with a fork. Add the lemon juice, salt, and pepper to taste. Spread the avocado mixture evenly over the toasted bread.
3. **Poach the Egg:**
   - Fill a small saucepan with water and bring it to a gentle simmer. Crack the egg into a small bowl. Create a gentle whirlpool in the water with a spoon and carefully slide the egg into the center. Poach the egg for about 3-4 minutes until the white is set but the yolk remains runny. Remove with a slotted spoon and place it on top of the avocado toast.
4. **Season and Serve:**
   - Sprinkle additional salt and pepper over the egg, if desired. Serve immediately and enjoy your delicious and nutritious breakfast.

Macronutrients (approximate values):
- **Calories:** 300 kcal
- **Carbohydrates:** 25g
- **Fat:** 18g; **Protein:** 12g

Banana and Almond Butter Smoothie

Preparation Time: 5 minutes
Cooking Time: 0 minutes
Servings: 1 person
Ingredients:
- 1 large banana
- 1 tablespoon almond butter
- 1 cup almond milk (unsweetened)
- 1/2 teaspoon vanilla extract
- 1 teaspoon honey (optional)

Procedure:
1. **Prepare the Ingredients:**
   - Peel the banana and break it into chunks.
2. **Blend the Smoothie:**
   - In a blender, combine the banana chunks, almond butter, almond milk, vanilla extract, and honey (if using).
3. **Blend Until Smooth:**
   - Blend the ingredients on high speed until smooth and creamy, ensuring there are no lumps.
4. **Serve:**
   - Pour the smoothie into a glass and enjoy immediately.

Macronutrients (approximate values):
- **Calories:** 280 kcal
- **Carbohydrates:** 40g
- **Fat:** 12g
- **Protein:** 6g

Blueberry Oatmeal with Walnuts

Preparation Time: 5 minutes
Cooking Time: 10 minutes
Servings: 1 person
Ingredients:
- 1/2 cup rolled oats
- 1 cup water or milk (almond milk, if preferred)
- 1/2 cup fresh or frozen blueberries
- 1 tablespoon chopped walnuts
- 1 teaspoon honey or maple syrup (optional)

Procedure:
1. **Cook the Oats:**
   - In a small saucepan, bring the water or milk to a boil. Add the rolled oats and reduce the heat to a simmer. Cook for about 5-7 minutes, stirring occasionally, until the oats are soft and have absorbed most of the liquid.
2. **Add the Blueberries:**
   - Stir in the blueberries and continue to cook for another 2-3 minutes until the blueberries are warm and starting to burst.
3. **Serve:**
   - Pour the oatmeal into a bowl.
4. **Top and Sweeten:**
   - Sprinkle the chopped walnuts on top and drizzle with honey or maple syrup if desired. Serve immediately.

Macronutrients (approximate values):
- **Calories:** 300 kcal
- **Carbohydrates:** 45g
- **Fat:** 10g
- **Protein:** 7g

Greek Yogurt Parfait with Granola and Honey

Preparation Time: 5 minutes
Cooking Time: None
Servings: 1 person
Ingredients:

- 1 cup Greek yogurt
- 1/4 cup granola
- 1 tablespoon honey
- 1/2 cup mixed berries (e.g., blueberries, strawberries, raspberries)
- 1 tablespoon chopped nuts (optional)

Procedure:

1. **Layer the Yogurt:**
   - In a tall glass or bowl, add half of the Greek yogurt as the base layer.
2. **Add the Berries:**
   - Layer half of the mixed berries over the yogurt.
3. **Top with Granola and Honey:**
   - Sprinkle half of the granola on top of the berries, then drizzle with half of the honey.
4. **Repeat and Finish:**
   - Add the remaining yogurt, then top with the rest of the berries, granola, and a final drizzle of honey. If desired, sprinkle with chopped nuts for added crunch and nutrients. Serve immediately.

Macronutrients (approximate values):

- **Calories:** 350 kcal
- **Carbohydrates:** 45g
- **Fat:** 10g; **Protein:** 20g

Nutty Banana Pancakes

Preparation Time: 10 minutes
Cooking Time: 10 minutes
Servings: 1 person
Ingredients:

- 1 ripe banana, mashed
- 1 egg
- 1/4 cup almond flour
- 1/4 teaspoon baking powder
- 1 tablespoon chopped nuts (e.g., walnuts or almonds)

Procedure:

1. **Prepare the Batter:**
   - In a bowl, combine the mashed banana and egg, mixing until well blended.
   - Add the almond flour and baking powder to the banana mixture and stir until you have a smooth batter. Fold in the chopped nuts.
2. **Heat the Pan:**
   - Preheat a non-stick skillet or griddle over medium heat. Lightly grease with cooking spray or a small amount of oil if necessary.
3. **Cook the Pancakes:**
   - Pour small amounts of the batter onto the skillet to form pancakes (about 2-3 inches in diameter). Cook until bubbles start to form on the surface and the edges look set, about 2-3 minutes. Flip and cook for an additional 2-3 minutes on the other side until golden brown.
4. **Serve:**
   - Serve the pancakes warm. Optionally, top with a drizzle of honey or a few additional nuts for extra flavor and texture.

Macronutrients (approximate values):

- **Calories:** 300 kcal
- **Carbohydrates:** 30g
- **Fat:** 15g
- **Protein:** 12g

Overnight Chia Pudding with Mixed Nuts

Preparation Time: 5 minutes
Cooking Time: None (overnight refrigeration)
Servings: 1 person
Ingredients:
- 3 tablespoons chia seeds
- 1 cup unsweetened almond milk
- 1 teaspoon honey or maple syrup
- 2 tablespoons mixed nuts (e.g., almonds, walnuts, pecans), chopped
- 1/4 teaspoon vanilla extract (optional)

Procedure:
1. **Combine Ingredients:**
    - In a jar or bowl, mix the chia seeds, almond milk, honey or maple syrup, and vanilla extract (if using). Stir well to combine.
2. **Refrigerate:**
    - Cover the jar or bowl and refrigerate overnight or for at least 4 hours, allowing the chia seeds to absorb the liquid and form a pudding-like consistency.
3. **Stir and Adjust:**
    - In the morning, stir the chia pudding to ensure even texture. If it's too thick, you can add a little more almond milk until you reach your desired consistency.
4. **Serve:**
    - Top the chia pudding with the chopped mixed nuts just before serving. Enjoy your delicious and nutritious breakfast!

Macronutrients (approximate values):
- **Calories:** 350 kcal
- **Carbohydrates:** 30g
- **Fat:** 20g
- **Protein:** 10g

Quinoa Breakfast Bowl with Spinach and Avocados

Preparation Time: 10 minutes
Cooking Time: 15 minutes
Servings: 1 person
Ingredients:
- 1/2 cup quinoa, rinsed
- 1 cup fresh spinach leaves
- 1/2 avocado, sliced
- 1 tablespoon olive oil
- Salt and pepper to taste

Procedure:
1. **Cook Quinoa:**
    - In a small pot, bring 1 cup of water to a boil. Add the rinsed quinoa, reduce the heat to low, cover, and simmer for about 15 minutes or until the water is absorbed and the quinoa is fluffy.
2. **Sauté Spinach:**
    - While the quinoa is cooking, heat the olive oil in a pan over medium heat. Add the spinach leaves and sauté until wilted, about 2-3 minutes. Season with a pinch of salt and pepper.
3. **Assemble the Bowl:**
    - Once the quinoa is cooked, transfer it to a bowl. Top with the sautéed spinach and sliced avocado.
4. **Season and Serve:**
    - Drizzle a little more olive oil on top if desired and season with additional salt and pepper to taste. Serve immediately and enjoy your nutritious and delicious breakfast bowl!

Macronutrients (approximate values):
- **Calories:** 400 kcal
- **Carbohydrates:** 40g
- **Fat:** 22g
- **Protein:** 10g

Salmon and Cream Cheese Bagel

Preparation Time: 5 minutes
Cooking Time: 0 minutes
Servings: 1 person
Ingredients:
- 1 whole grain bagel, sliced and toasted
- 2 tablespoons cream cheese
- 2 ounces smoked salmon
- 1 tablespoon capers
- 1 tablespoon thinly sliced red onion

Procedure:
1. **Prepare the Bagel:**
   - Slice the whole grain bagel in half and toast it to your desired level of crispness.
2. **Spread the Cream Cheese:**
   - Once the bagel is toasted, spread 1 tablespoon of cream cheese on each half of the bagel.
3. **Add the Salmon:**
   - Layer 1 ounce of smoked salmon on top of the cream cheese on each half of the bagel.
4. **Top with Capers and Onion:**
   - Sprinkle the capers evenly over the smoked salmon, and add the thinly sliced red onion on top. Serve immediately and enjoy!

Macronutrients (approximate values):
- **Calories:** 380 kcal
- **Carbohydrates:** 40g
- **Fat:** 18g
- **Protein:** 18g

Scrambled Eggs with Smoked Salmon and Spinach

Preparation Time: 5 minutes
Cooking Time: 5 minutes
Servings: 1 person
Ingredients:
- 2 large eggs
- 1/4 cup smoked salmon, chopped
- 1/2 cup fresh spinach, chopped
- 1 tablespoon olive oil
- Salt and pepper to taste

Procedure:
1. **Prepare the Ingredients:**
   - Crack the eggs into a bowl and whisk until well combined. Season with a pinch of salt and pepper.
2. **Cook the Spinach:**
   - Heat the olive oil in a non-stick skillet over medium heat. Add the chopped spinach and sauté until wilted, about 1-2 minutes.
3. **Add the Eggs and Salmon:**
   - Pour the beaten eggs into the skillet with the spinach. Add the chopped smoked salmon. Stir gently and continuously to scramble the eggs, cooking until they reach your desired level of doneness, about 2-3 minutes.
4. **Serve:**
   - Transfer the scrambled eggs with smoked salmon and spinach to a plate. Serve immediately and enjoy!

Macronutrients (approximate values):
- **Calories:** 280 kcal
- **Carbohydrates:** 2g
- **Fat:** 22g
- **Protein:** 20g

Sweet Potato and Black Bean Breakfast Burrito

Preparation Time: 10 minutes
Cooking Time: 15 minutes
Servings: 1 person
Ingredients:
- 1 medium sweet potato, peeled and diced
- 1/2 cup black beans, drained and rinsed
- 1 large whole wheat tortilla
- 1 tablespoon olive oil
- 1/4 cup shredded cheddar cheese
- Salt and pepper to taste

Procedure:
1. **Cook the Sweet Potato:**
   - Heat the olive oil in a skillet over medium heat. Add the diced sweet potato and cook until tender, about 10-12 minutes, stirring occasionally. Season with salt and pepper to taste.
2. **Add the Black Beans:**
   - Once the sweet potatoes are cooked, add the black beans to the skillet. Stir to combine and cook for another 2-3 minutes until heated through.
3. **Assemble the Burrito:**
   - Lay the whole wheat tortilla flat on a plate. Sprinkle the shredded cheddar cheese in the center of the tortilla. Add the sweet potato and black bean mixture on top of the cheese.
4. **Wrap and Serve:**
   - Fold the sides of the tortilla over the filling, then roll it up tightly into a burrito. Serve immediately and enjoy!

Macronutrients (approximate values):
- **Calories:** 350 kcal
- **Carbohydrates:** 48g
- **Fat:** 14g
- **Protein:** 12g

High-Calorie Lunch Recipes

Avocado Chicken Salad

Preparation Time: 10 minutes
Cooking Time: 15 minutes
Servings: 1 person
Ingredients:
- 1 cooked chicken breast, shredded
- 1/2 avocado, diced
- 1/4 cup cherry tomatoes, halved
- 1 tablespoon olive oil
- Salt and pepper to taste

Procedure:
1. **Combine Ingredients:**
   - In a bowl, combine shredded chicken, diced avocado, and cherry tomatoes.
2. **Dress the Salad:**
   - Drizzle with olive oil, and season with salt and pepper. Toss gently to combine.
3. **Serve:**
   - Serve immediately and enjoy!

Macronutrients (approximate values):
- **Calories:** 400 kcal
- **Carbohydrates:** 10g
- **Fat:** 28g
- **Protein:** 25g

Beef and Sweet Potato Stew

Preparation Time: 10 minutes
Cooking Time: 40 minutes
Servings: 1 person
Ingredients:
- 150g beef stew meat, diced
- 1 medium sweet potato, peeled and diced
- 1/2 cup beef broth
- 1 tablespoon olive oil
- Salt and pepper to taste

Procedure:
1. **Cook Beef:**
   - In a pot, heat olive oil over medium heat. Add beef and cook until browned.
2. **Add Sweet Potatoes:**
   - Add sweet potatoes and beef broth. Bring to a boil, then reduce heat and simmer for 30 minutes or until sweet potatoes are tender.
3. **Season and Serve:**
   - Season with salt and pepper. Serve hot.

Macronutrients (approximate values):
- **Calories:** 450 kcal
- **Carbohydrates:** 30g
- **Fat:** 20g
- **Protein:** 35g

Chicken Pesto Pasta

Preparation Time: 10 minutes
Cooking Time: 15 minutes
Servings: 1 person
Ingredients:
- 1 cup cooked whole wheat pasta
- 1 cooked chicken breast, sliced
- 2 tablespoons pesto
- 1/4 cup cherry tomatoes, halved
- 1 tablespoon olive oil

Procedure:
1. **Prepare Pasta:**
   - Cook pasta according to package instructions.
2. **Combine Ingredients:**
   - In a bowl, combine cooked pasta, sliced chicken, pesto, and cherry tomatoes.
3. **Serve:**
   - Drizzle with olive oil, toss to combine, and serve immediately.

Macronutrients (approximate values):
- **Calories:** 500 kcal
- **Carbohydrates:** 50g
- **Fat:** 25g
- **Protein:** 30g

Grilled Cheese and Tomato Soup

Preparation Time: 10 minutes
Cooking Time: 20 minutes
Servings: 1 person
Ingredients:
- 2 slices whole grain bread
- 2 slices cheddar cheese
- 1 cup tomato soup
- 1 tablespoon butter

Procedure:
1. **Make Grilled Cheese:**
   - Butter one side of each bread slice. Place cheese between the unbuttered sides and grill in a pan until golden brown.
2. **Heat Soup:**
   - Heat tomato soup in a pot until hot.
3. **Serve:**
   - Serve grilled cheese with hot tomato soup.

Macronutrients (approximate values):
- **Calories:** 600 kcal
- **Carbohydrates:** 50g
- **Fat:** 30g
- **Protein:** 25g

Lentil and Quinoa Salad with Feta

Preparation Time: 10 minutes
Cooking Time: 20 minutes
Servings: 1 person
Ingredients:
- 1/2 cup cooked lentils
- 1/2 cup cooked quinoa
- 1/4 cup crumbled feta cheese
- 1/4 cup diced cucumber
- 1 tablespoon olive oil

Procedure:
1. **Combine Ingredients:**
   - In a bowl, combine lentils, quinoa, feta cheese, and cucumber.
2. **Dress the Salad:**
   - Drizzle with olive oil and toss to combine.
3. **Serve:**
   - Serve immediately and enjoy.

Macronutrients (approximate values):
- **Calories:** 450 kcal
- **Carbohydrates:** 50g
- **Fat:** 20g
- **Protein:** 20g

Salmon and Avocado Rice Bowl

Preparation Time: 10 minutes
Cooking Time: 15 minutes
Servings: 1 person
Ingredients:

- 1/2 cup cooked brown rice
- 1 cooked salmon fillet, flaked
- 1/2 avocado, sliced
- 1 tablespoon soy sauce

Procedure:

1. **Prepare Rice:**
   - Cook brown rice according to package instructions.
2. **Assemble Bowl:**
   - In a bowl, combine cooked rice, flaked salmon, and avocado slices.
3. **Serve:**
   - Drizzle with soy sauce and serve.

Macronutrients (approximate values):

- **Calories:** 500 kcal
- **Carbohydrates:** 45g
- **Fat:** 25g
- **Protein:** 30g

Shrimp and Avocado Tacos

Preparation Time: 10 minutes
Cooking Time: 10 minutes
Servings: 1 person
Ingredients:

- 100g shrimp, peeled and deveined
- 1/2 avocado, sliced
- 2 whole wheat tortillas
- 1 tablespoon olive oil

Procedure:

1. **Cook Shrimp:**
   - Heat olive oil in a pan over medium heat. Cook shrimp until pink and cooked through.
2. **Assemble Tacos:**
   - Place shrimp and avocado slices on tortillas.
3. **Serve:**
   - Serve immediately and enjoy.

Macronutrients (approximate values):

- **Calories:** 450 kcal
- **Carbohydrates:** 35g
- **Fat:** 25g
- **Protein:** 20g

Spinach and Ricotta Stuffed Chicken Breast

Preparation Time: 10 minutes
Cooking Time: 25 minutes
Servings: 1 person
Ingredients:
- 1 chicken breast, butterflied
- 1/2 cup spinach, wilted
- 1/4 cup ricotta cheese
- 1 tablespoon olive oil

Procedure:
1. **Prepare Filling:**
    - Mix wilted spinach and ricotta cheese.
2. **Stuff Chicken:**
    - Stuff the chicken breast with the spinach and ricotta mixture. Secure with toothpicks.
3. **Cook Chicken:**
    - Heat olive oil in a pan over medium heat. Cook the chicken until cooked through, about 25 minutes.

Macronutrients (approximate values):
- **Calories:** 400 kcal
- **Carbohydrates:** 5g
- **Fat:** 20g
- **Protein:** 45g

Turkey and Hummus Wrap

Preparation Time: 10 minutes
Cooking Time: None
Servings: 1 person
Ingredients:
- 1 whole wheat tortilla
- 3 slices turkey breast
- 2 tablespoons hummus
- 1/4 cup shredded lettuce

Procedure:
1. **Assemble Wrap:**
    - Spread hummus on the tortilla. Layer with turkey slices and shredded lettuce.
2. **Roll Up:**
    - Roll up the tortilla tightly.
3. **Serve:**
    - Serve immediately and enjoy.

Macronutrients (approximate values):
- **Calories:** 350 kcal
- **Carbohydrates:** 35g
- **Fat:** 10g
- **Protein:** 25g

Veggie and Hummus Wrap

Preparation Time: 10 minutes
Cooking Time: None
Servings: 1 person
Ingredients:
- 1 whole wheat tortilla
- 2 tablespoons hummus
- 1/4 cup shredded carrots
- 1/4 cup cucumber slices
- 1/4 cup bell pepper slices

Procedure:
1. **Assemble Wrap:**
   - Spread hummus on the tortilla. Layer with shredded carrots, cucumber slices, and bell pepper slices.
2. **Roll Up:**
   - Roll up the tortilla tightly.
3. **Serve:**
   - Serve immediately and enjoy.

Macronutrients (approximate values):
- **Calories:** 300 kcal
- **Carbohydrates:** 40g
- **Fat:** 10g
- **Protein:** 10g

High-Calorie Dinner Recipes

Baked Salmon with Quinoa and Veggies

Preparation Time: 15 minutes
Cooking Time: 30 minutes
Servings: 1 person
Ingredients:
- 1 salmon fillet
- 1/2 cup cooked quinoa
- 1/2 cup mixed vegetables (e.g., bell peppers, zucchini)
- 1 tablespoon olive oil
- Salt and pepper to taste

Procedure:
1. **Preheat Oven:**
   - Preheat the oven to 375°F (190°C).
2. **Prepare Salmon:**
   - Place the salmon fillet on a baking sheet. Drizzle with olive oil, and season with salt and pepper.
3. **Bake Salmon:**
   - Bake the salmon for 20-25 minutes until cooked through.
4. **Serve:**
   - Serve the salmon with cooked quinoa and sautéed mixed vegetables.

Macronutrients (approximate values):
- **Calories:** 600 kcal
- **Carbohydrates:** 45g
- **Fat:** 30g
- **Protein:** 35g

Beef Stir-Fry with Broccoli

Preparation Time: 10 minutes
Cooking Time: 15 minutes
Servings: 1 person
Ingredients:
- 150g beef strips
- 1 cup broccoli florets
- 1 tablespoon soy sauce
- 1 tablespoon olive oil
- 1/4 cup sliced onions

Procedure:
1. **Heat Oil:**
   - Heat olive oil in a pan over medium-high heat.
2. **Cook Beef:**
   - Add beef strips and cook until browned.
3. **Add Veggies:**
   - Add broccoli and onions. Stir-fry for 5 minutes, then add soy sauce.
4. **Serve:**
   - Serve hot and enjoy.

Macronutrients (approximate values):
- **Calories:** 500 kcal
- **Carbohydrates:** 20g
- **Fat:** 30g
- **Protein:** 35g

Chicken Alfredo with Zoodles

Preparation Time: 10 minutes
Cooking Time: 20 minutes
Servings: 1 person
Ingredients:
- 1 chicken breast, sliced
- 1 zucchini, spiralized into noodles
- 1/2 cup Alfredo sauce
- 1 tablespoon olive oil
- 1 garlic clove, minced

Procedure:
1. **Cook Chicken:**
   - Heat olive oil in a pan and cook chicken slices until browned.
2. **Add Garlic:**
   - Add minced garlic and cook for 1 minute.
3. **Combine Ingredients:**
   - Add zucchini noodles and Alfredo sauce. Cook for 3-4 minutes.
4. **Serve:**
   - Serve immediately and enjoy.

Macronutrients (approximate values):
- **Calories:** 550 kcal
- **Carbohydrates:** 15g
- **Fat:** 35g
- **Protein:** 40g

Grilled Lamb Chops with Sweet Potato Mash

Preparation Time: 10 minutes
Cooking Time: 25 minutes
Servings: 1 person
Ingredients:
- 2 lamb chops
- 1 sweet potato, peeled and cubed
- 1 tablespoon olive oil
- Salt and pepper to taste
- 1 tablespoon butter

Procedure:
1. **Cook Sweet Potato:**
   - Boil sweet potato cubes until tender, then mash with butter.
2. **Season Lamb Chops:**
   - Season lamb chops with salt and pepper.
3. **Grill Lamb Chops:**
   - Grill lamb chops for 5-6 minutes per side until desired doneness.
4. **Serve:**
   - Serve lamb chops with sweet potato mash.

Macronutrients (approximate values):
- **Calories:** 650 kcal
- **Carbohydrates:** 45g
- **Fat:** 35g
- **Protein:** 35g

Lentil and Vegetable Casserole

Preparation Time: 15 minutes
Cooking Time: 40 minutes
Servings: 1 person
Ingredients:
- 1 cup cooked lentils
- 1/2 cup diced carrots
- 1/2 cup diced celery
- 1/4 cup diced onions
- 1 tablespoon olive oil

Procedure:
1. **Preheat Oven:**
   - Preheat oven to 350°F (175°C).
2. **Sauté Veggies:**
   - Sauté carrots, celery, and onions in olive oil until tender.
3. **Combine Ingredients:**
   - Combine cooked lentils and sautéed veggies in a baking dish.
4. **Bake:**
   - Bake for 30 minutes until heated through.

Macronutrients (approximate values):
- **Calories:** 450 kcal
- **Carbohydrates:** 60g
- **Fat:** 10g
- **Protein:** 20g

Pork Tenderloin with Apple and Sage

Preparation Time: 10 minutes
Cooking Time: 25 minutes
Servings: 1 person
Ingredients:
- 1 pork tenderloin
- 1 apple, sliced
- 1 tablespoon olive oil
- 1 tablespoon fresh sage, chopped
- Salt and pepper to taste

Procedure:
1. **Preheat Oven:**
   - Preheat oven to 375°F (190°C).
2. **Season Pork:**
   - Season pork tenderloin with salt, pepper, and chopped sage.
3. **Cook Pork:**
   - In a skillet, heat olive oil and brown pork tenderloin on all sides.
4. **Bake:**
   - Transfer pork to a baking dish, add apple slices, and bake for 20 minutes.

Macronutrients (approximate values):
- **Calories:** 500 kcal
- **Carbohydrates:** 30g
- **Fat:** 20g
- **Protein:** 50g

Quinoa-Stuffed Portobello Mushrooms

Preparation Time: 10 minutes
Cooking Time: 20 minutes
Servings: 1 person
Ingredients:
- 2 large portobello mushrooms
- 1/2 cup cooked quinoa
- 1/4 cup diced bell peppers
- 1 tablespoon olive oil
- Salt and pepper to taste

Procedure:
1. **Preheat Oven:**
   - Preheat oven to 375°F (190°C).
2. **Prepare Filling:**
   - Mix cooked quinoa and diced bell peppers. Season with salt and pepper.
3. **Stuff Mushrooms:**
   - Stuff the mushrooms with the quinoa mixture and drizzle with olive oil.
4. **Bake:**
   - Bake for 20 minutes until mushrooms are tender.

Macronutrients (approximate values):
- **Calories:** 400 kcal
- **Carbohydrates:** 50g
- **Fat:** 15g
- **Protein:** 15g

Shrimp and Avocado Salad

Preparation Time: 10 minutes
Cooking Time: 10 minutes
Servings: 1 person
Ingredients:
- 100g shrimp, peeled and deveined
- 1/2 avocado, sliced
- 2 cups mixed greens
- 1 tablespoon olive oil
- 1 tablespoon lemon juice

Procedure:
1. **Cook Shrimp:**
   - Heat olive oil in a pan and cook shrimp until pink and cooked through.
2. **Prepare Salad:**
   - In a bowl, combine mixed greens, avocado slices, and cooked shrimp.
3. **Dress Salad:**
   - Drizzle with lemon juice and toss gently.
4. **Serve:**
   - Serve immediately.

Macronutrients (approximate values):
- **Calories:** 450 kcal
- **Carbohydrates:** 15g
- **Fat:** 30g
- **Protein:** 25g

Spaghetti Squash with Meatballs

Preparation Time: 10 minutes
Cooking Time: 40 minutes
Servings: 1 person
Ingredients:
- 1 small spaghetti squash
- 4 meatballs (pre-cooked or homemade)
- 1 cup marinara sauce
- 1 tablespoon olive oil
- Salt and pepper to taste

Procedure:
1. **Cook Spaghetti Squash:**
   - Cut the squash in half, remove seeds, and bake at 375°F (190°C) for 40 minutes.
2. **Prepare Meatballs:**
   - Heat meatballs and marinara sauce in a pan.
3. **Combine:**
   - Scrape out spaghetti squash strands and mix with meatballs and sauce.
4. **Serve:**
   - Season with salt and pepper and serve hot.

Macronutrients (approximate values):
- **Calories:** 500 kcal
- **Carbohydrates:** 45g
- **Fat:** 20g
- **Protein:** 25g

Stuffed Bell Peppers with Ground Turkey

Preparation Time: 15 minutes
Cooking Time: 30 minutes
Servings: 1 person
Ingredients:
- 2 bell peppers, tops cut off and seeds removed
- 150g ground turkey
- 1/2 cup cooked brown rice
- 1/4 cup diced tomatoes
- 1 tablespoon olive oil

Procedure:
1. **Preheat Oven:**
    - Preheat oven to 375°F (190°C).
2. **Prepare Filling:**
    - Cook ground turkey in olive oil until browned, then mix with cooked rice and diced tomatoes.
3. **Stuff Peppers:**
    - Stuff bell peppers with the turkey mixture.
4. **Bake:**
    - Place stuffed peppers in a baking dish and bake for 30 minutes.

Macronutrients (approximate values):
- **Calories:** 500 kcal
- **Carbohydrates:** 40g
- **Fat:** 20g
- **Protein:** 35g

High-Calorie Snacks and Desserts recipes

Almond Butter Energy Balls

Preparation Time: 15 minutes
Cooking Time: None
Servings: 1 person
Ingredients:
- 1/2 cup almond butter
- 1/2 cup rolled oats
- 1/4 cup honey
- 1/4 cup chocolate chips
- 1 tablespoon chia seeds

Procedure:
1. **Mix Ingredients:**
    - In a bowl, combine almond butter, rolled oats, honey, chocolate chips, and chia seeds.
2. **Form Balls:**
    - Roll mixture into small balls using your hands.
3. **Chill:**
    - Refrigerate for at least 30 minutes.
4. **Serve:**
    - Enjoy as a quick, high-calorie snack.

Macronutrients (approximate values per serving):
- **Calories:** 400 kcal
- **Carbohydrates:** 45g
- **Fat:** 20g
- **Protein:** 10g

Avocado Chocolate Mousse

Preparation Time: 10 minutes
Cooking Time: None
Servings: 1 person
Ingredients:
- 1 ripe avocado
- 2 tablespoons cocoa powder
- 2 tablespoons honey
- 1/2 teaspoon vanilla extract
- Pinch of salt

Procedure:
1. **Blend Ingredients:**
   - Combine all ingredients in a blender until smooth.
2. **Chill:**
   - Refrigerate for at least 30 minutes to set.
3. **Serve:**
   - Serve chilled.

Macronutrients (approximate values per serving):
- **Calories:** 300 kcal
- **Carbohydrates:** 35g
- **Fat:** 20g
- **Protein:** 3g

Banana Walnut Bread

Preparation Time: 10 minutes
Cooking Time: 45 minutes
Servings: 1 person
Ingredients:
- 1 ripe banana
- 1/2 cup whole wheat flour
- 1/4 cup walnuts, chopped
- 1/4 cup honey
- 1 egg

Procedure:
1. **Preheat Oven:**
   - Preheat the oven to 350°F (175°C).
2. **Mix Ingredients:**
   - In a bowl, mash the banana and mix in the flour, walnuts, honey, and egg until well combined.
3. **Bake:**
   - Pour batter into a greased loaf pan and bake for 45 minutes.
4. **Serve:**
   - Let cool before serving.

Macronutrients (approximate values per serving):
- **Calories:** 400 kcal
- **Carbohydrates:** 55g
- **Fat:** 15g
- **Protein:** 7g

Dark Chocolate Almond Bark

Preparation Time: 5 minutes
Cooking Time: 10 minutes
Servings: 1 person
Ingredients:
- 1/2 cup dark chocolate chips
- 1/4 cup almonds, chopped
- 1 tablespoon coconut oil
- Pinch of sea salt

Procedure:
1. **Melt Chocolate:**
    - Melt dark chocolate chips and coconut oil in a microwave-safe bowl.
2. **Mix In Almonds:**
    - Stir in chopped almonds.
3. **Spread and Chill:**
    - Spread mixture onto a baking sheet and sprinkle with sea salt. Refrigerate until set.
4. **Serve:**
    - Break into pieces and enjoy.

Macronutrients (approximate values per serving):
- **Calories:** 350 kcal
- **Carbohydrates:** 30g
- **Fat:** 25g
- **Protein:** 5g

Greek Yogurt with Honey and Granola

Preparation Time: 5 minutes
Cooking Time: None
Servings: 1 person
Ingredients:
- 1 cup Greek yogurt
- 2 tablespoons honey
- 1/4 cup granola
- 1/4 cup mixed berries

Procedure:
1. **Layer Yogurt:**
    - In a bowl, layer Greek yogurt and honey.
2. **Add Toppings:**
    - Top with granola and mixed berries.
3. **Serve:**
    - Enjoy immediately.

Macronutrients (approximate values per serving):
- **Calories:** 400 kcal
- **Carbohydrates:** 50g
- **Fat:** 10g
- **Protein:** 20g

Nutty Apple Slices

Preparation Time: 5 minutes
Cooking Time: None
Servings: 1 person
Ingredients:
- 1 apple, sliced
- 2 tablespoons almond butter
- 1 tablespoon chopped nuts (e.g., walnuts, pecans)

Procedure:
1. **Prepare Apple:**
    - Slice the apple into thin rounds.
2. **Spread Almond Butter:**
    - Spread almond butter on each apple slice.
3. **Add Nuts:**
    - Sprinkle chopped nuts on top.
4. **Serve:**
    - Enjoy immediately.

Macronutrients (approximate values per serving):
- **Calories:** 300 kcal
- **Carbohydrates:** 40g
- **Fat:** 15g
- **Protein:** 5g

Oatmeal Raisin Cookies

Preparation Time: 10 minutes
Cooking Time: 15 minutes
Servings: 1 person
Ingredients:
- 1/2 cup rolled oats
- 1/4 cup raisins
- 1/4 cup whole wheat flour
- 1/4 cup honey
- 1 egg

Procedure:
1. **Preheat Oven:**
    - Preheat oven to 350°F (175°C).
2. **Mix Ingredients:**
    - Combine oats, raisins, flour, honey, and egg in a bowl.
3. **Bake:**
    - Drop spoonfuls of dough onto a baking sheet and bake for 15 minutes.
4. **Serve:**
    - Let cool before serving.

Macronutrients (approximate values per serving):
- **Calories:** 350 kcal
- **Carbohydrates:** 60g
- **Fat:** 10g
- **Protein:** 6g

Peanut Butter and Banana Toast

Preparation Time: 5 minutes
Cooking Time: None
Servings: 1 person
Ingredients:
- 1 slice whole grain bread
- 1 tablespoon peanut butter
- 1/2 banana, sliced
- 1 teaspoon honey

Procedure:
1. **Toast Bread:**
    - Toast the slice of whole grain bread.
2. **Spread Peanut Butter:**
    - Spread peanut butter on the toast.
3. **Add Banana:**
    - Top with banana slices and drizzle with honey.
4. **Serve:**
    - Enjoy immediately.

Macronutrients (approximate values per serving):
- **Calories:** 350 kcal
- **Carbohydrates:** 45g
- **Fat:** 15g
- **Protein:** 8g

Protein-Packed Smoothie Bowl

Preparation Time: 10 minutes
Cooking Time: None
Servings: 1 person
Ingredients:
- 1 scoop protein powder
- 1/2 banana
- 1/2 cup Greek yogurt
- 1/4 cup granola
- 1/4 cup mixed berries

Procedure:
1. **Blend Smoothie:**
    - Blend protein powder, banana, and Greek yogurt until smooth.
2. **Pour into Bowl:**
    - Pour the smoothie mixture into a bowl.
3. **Add Toppings:**
    - Top with granola and mixed berries.
4. **Serve:**
    - Enjoy immediately.

Macronutrients (approximate values per serving):
- **Calories:** 400 kcal
- **Carbohydrates:** 40g
- **Fat:** 10g
- **Protein:** 30g

Sweet Potato Brownies

Preparation Time: 10 minutes
Cooking Time: 25 minutes
Servings: 1 person
Ingredients:
- 1/2 cup mashed sweet potato
- 1/4 cup cocoa powder
- 1/4 cup almond butter
- 1/4 cup honey
- 1 egg

Procedure:
1. **Preheat Oven:**
    - Preheat oven to 350°F (175°C).
2. **Mix Ingredients:**
    - Combine mashed sweet potato, cocoa powder, almond butter, honey, and egg in a bowl.
3. **Bake:**
    - Pour batter into a greased baking dish and bake for 25 minutes.
4. **Serve:**
    - Let cool before serving.

Macronutrients (approximate values per serving):
- **Calories:** 350 kcal
- **Carbohydrates:** 45g
- **Fat:** 15g
- **Protein:** 8g

Plant-Based Recipes

Avocado and Black Bean Salad

Preparation Time: 10 minutes
Cooking Time: None
Servings: 1 person
Ingredients:
- 1 avocado, diced
- 1/2 cup black beans, rinsed and drained
- 1/2 cup cherry tomatoes, halved
- 1 tablespoon lime juice
- 1 tablespoon chopped cilantro

Procedure:
1. **Combine Ingredients:**
    - In a bowl, mix diced avocado, black beans, and cherry tomatoes.
2. **Add Lime Juice:**
    - Drizzle with lime juice and toss to combine.
3. **Add Cilantro:**
    - Sprinkle chopped cilantro on top.
4. **Serve:**
    - Serve immediately and enjoy.

Macronutrients (approximate values per serving):
- **Calories:** 300 kcal
- **Carbohydrates:** 30g
- **Fat:** 18g
- **Protein:** 8g

Cauliflower Buffalo Wings

Preparation Time: 10 minutes
Cooking Time: 25 minutes
Servings: 1 person
Ingredients:
- 1 small head cauliflower, cut into florets
- 1/2 cup whole wheat flour
- 1/2 cup water
- 1/2 cup hot sauce
- 1 tablespoon olive oil

Procedure:
1. **Preheat Oven:**
   - Preheat oven to 450°F (230°C).
2. **Mix Batter:**
   - In a bowl, combine flour and water to make a batter. Toss cauliflower florets in the batter until well coated.
3. **Bake:**
   - Spread coated florets on a baking sheet and bake for 20 minutes. Toss with hot sauce and olive oil, then bake for an additional 5 minutes.
4. **Serve:**
   - Serve with your favorite dipping sauce.

Macronutrients (approximate values per serving):
- **Calories:** 250 kcal
- **Carbohydrates:** 40g
- **Fat:** 8g
- **Protein:** 6g

Chickpea and Spinach Curry

Preparation Time: 10 minutes
Cooking Time: 20 minutes
Servings: 1 person
Ingredients:
- 1/2 cup chickpeas, rinsed and drained
- 1 cup spinach
- 1/2 cup coconut milk
- 1 tablespoon curry powder
- 1 teaspoon olive oil

Procedure:
1. **Sauté Spinach:**
   - In a pan, heat olive oil and sauté spinach until wilted.
2. **Add Chickpeas and Curry Powder:**
   - Add chickpeas and curry powder, stir well.
3. **Add Coconut Milk:**
   - Pour in coconut milk and simmer for 10 minutes.
4. **Serve:**
   - Serve hot with brown rice or quinoa.

Macronutrients (approximate values per serving):
- **Calories:** 300 kcal
- **Carbohydrates:** 30g
- **Fat:** 16g
- **Protein:** 10g

Grilled Portobello Mushrooms with Quinoa

Preparation Time: 10 minutes
Cooking Time: 20 minutes
Servings: 1 person
Ingredients:

- 2 portobello mushrooms
- 1/2 cup quinoa, cooked
- 1 tablespoon balsamic vinegar
- 1 teaspoon olive oil
- 1 clove garlic, minced

Procedure:

1. **Marinate Mushrooms:**
    - Marinate mushrooms with balsamic vinegar, olive oil, and minced garlic for 10 minutes.
2. **Grill Mushrooms:**
    - Grill mushrooms for 5-7 minutes on each side.
3. **Cook Quinoa:**
    - Cook quinoa according to package instructions.
4. **Serve:**
    - Serve grilled mushrooms on a bed of quinoa.

Macronutrients (approximate values per serving):

- **Calories:** 300 kcal
- **Carbohydrates:** 45g
- **Fat:** 8g
- **Protein:** 12g

Lentil and Vegetable Stew

Preparation Time: 10 minutes
Cooking Time: 30 minutes
Servings: 1 person
Ingredients:

- 1/2 cup lentils
- 1 carrot, chopped
- 1 celery stalk, chopped
- 1/2 onion, chopped
- 1 cup vegetable broth

Procedure:

1. **Sauté Vegetables:**
    - In a pot, sauté onion, carrot, and celery until tender.
2. **Add Lentils:**
    - Add lentils and vegetable broth. Bring to a boil.
3. **Simmer:**
    - Reduce heat and simmer for 30 minutes.
4. **Serve:**
    - Serve hot, garnished with fresh herbs if desired.

Macronutrients (approximate values per serving):

- **Calories:** 300 kcal
- **Carbohydrates:** 50g
- **Fat:** 3g
- **Protein:** 18g

Mixed Vegetable Stir-Fry with Tofu

Preparation Time: 10 minutes
Cooking Time: 15 minutes
Servings: 1 person
Ingredients:
- 1/2 cup tofu, cubed
- 1 cup mixed vegetables (bell peppers, broccoli, carrots)
- 1 tablespoon soy sauce
- 1 teaspoon olive oil
- 1 clove garlic, minced

Procedure:
1. **Sauté Garlic:**
    - In a pan, heat olive oil and sauté garlic until fragrant.
2. **Add Tofu:**
    - Add tofu and cook until golden brown.
3. **Add Vegetables:**
    - Add mixed vegetables and soy sauce. Stir-fry for 5-7 minutes.
4. **Serve:**
    - Serve hot over brown rice or noodles.

Macronutrients (approximate values per serving):
- **Calories:** 250 kcal
- **Carbohydrates:** 25g
- **Fat:** 12g
- **Protein:** 15g

Roasted Beet and Kale Salad

Preparation Time: 10 minutes
Cooking Time: 25 minutes
Servings: 1 person
Ingredients:
- 1 beet, roasted and sliced
- 1 cup kale, chopped
- 1 tablespoon olive oil
- 1 tablespoon balsamic vinegar
- 1 tablespoon sunflower seeds

Procedure:
1. **Roast Beet:**
    - Preheat oven to 400°F (200°C). Roast beet for 25 minutes, then slice.
2. **Massage Kale:**
    - Massage kale with olive oil and balsamic vinegar until tender.
3. **Add Beets:**
    - Add roasted beets to the kale.
4. **Serve:**
    - Sprinkle sunflower seeds on top and serve.

Macronutrients (approximate values per serving):
- **Calories:** 250 kcal
- **Carbohydrates:** 20g
- **Fat:** 16g
- **Protein:** 5g

Spaghetti Squash with Tomato Basil Sauce

Preparation Time: 10 minutes
Cooking Time: 40 minutes
Servings: 1 person
Ingredients:
- 1/2 spaghetti squash
- 1 cup tomato sauce
- 1/4 cup fresh basil, chopped
- 1 tablespoon olive oil
- 1 clove garlic, minced

Procedure:
1. **Cook Spaghetti Squash:**
   - Preheat oven to 400°F (200°C). Roast spaghetti squash for 40 minutes, then scrape out strands.
2. **Prepare Sauce:**
   - In a pan, heat olive oil and sauté garlic. Add tomato sauce and basil. Simmer for 10 minutes.
3. **Combine:**
   - Toss spaghetti squash strands with tomato basil sauce.
4. **Serve:**
   - Serve hot, garnished with additional basil if desired.

Macronutrients (approximate values per serving):
- **Calories:** 200 kcal
- **Carbohydrates:** 30g
- **Fat:** 10g
- **Protein:** 4g

Sweet Potato and Black Bean Tacos

Preparation Time: 10 minutes
Cooking Time: 20 minutes
Servings: 1 person
Ingredients:
- 1 small sweet potato, diced
- 1/2 cup black beans, rinsed and drained
- 1 small avocado, sliced
- 1 tablespoon olive oil
- 1 teaspoon taco seasoning

Procedure:
1. **Cook Sweet Potato:**
   - In a pan, heat olive oil and sauté sweet potato with taco seasoning until tender, about 15 minutes.
2. **Add Black Beans:**
   - Add black beans and cook for an additional 5 minutes.
3. **Prepare Tacos:**
   - Warm tortillas and fill with sweet potato and black bean mixture.
4. **Serve:**
   - Top with avocado slices and serve.

Macronutrients (approximate values per serving):
- **Calories:** 350 kcal
- **Carbohydrates:** 45g
- **Fat:** 15g
- **Protein:** 8g

Zucchini Noodles with Pesto

Preparation Time: 10 minutes
Cooking Time: 5 minutes
Servings: 1 person
Ingredients:
- 1 zucchini, spiralized
- 2 tablespoons pesto
- 1 tablespoon olive oil
- 1 tablespoon pine nuts
- 1 clove garlic, minced

Procedure:
1. **Sauté Garlic:**
   - In a pan, heat olive oil and sauté garlic until fragrant.
2. **Cook Zucchini:**
   - Add spiralized zucchini and cook for 3-5 minutes.
3. **Add Pesto:**
   - Toss zucchini noodles with pesto and pine nuts.
4. **Serve:**
   - Serve immediately.

Macronutrients (approximate values per serving):
- **Calories:** 300 kcal
- **Carbohydrates:** 10g
- **Fat:** 28g
- **Protein:** 4g

Vegan and vegetarian Protein Recipes

Black Bean and Corn Salad

Preparation Time: 10 minutes
Cooking Time: None
Servings: 1 person
Ingredients:
- 1/2 cup black beans, rinsed and drained
- 1/2 cup corn kernels
- 1/4 cup diced red bell pepper
- 1 tablespoon lime juice
- 1 tablespoon chopped cilantro

Procedure:
1. **Combine Ingredients:**
   - In a bowl, mix black beans, corn, and red bell pepper.
2. **Add Lime Juice:**
   - Drizzle with lime juice and toss to combine.
3. **Add Cilantro:**
   - Sprinkle chopped cilantro on top.
4. **Serve:**
   - Serve immediately.

Macronutrients (approximate values per serving):
- **Calories:** 220 kcal
- **Carbohydrates:** 40g
- **Fat:** 2g
- **Protein:** 10g

Chickpea and Spinach Stuffed Sweet Potatoes

Preparation Time: 10 minutes
Cooking Time: 40 minutes
Servings: 1 person
Ingredients:
- 1 medium sweet potato
- 1/2 cup chickpeas, rinsed and drained
- 1 cup spinach
- 1 tablespoon tahini
- 1 teaspoon olive oil

Procedure:
1. **Bake Sweet Potato:**
    - Preheat oven to 400°F (200°C). Pierce sweet potato with a fork and bake for 40 minutes until tender.
2. **Sauté Spinach:**
    - In a pan, heat olive oil and sauté spinach until wilted.
3. **Combine Chickpeas and Spinach:**
    - Mix chickpeas with sautéed spinach.
4. **Serve:**
    - Slice sweet potato and stuff with chickpea-spinach mixture. Drizzle with tahini before serving.

Macronutrients (approximate values per serving):
- **Calories:** 300 kcal
- **Carbohydrates:** 50g
- **Fat:** 10g
- **Protein:** 10g

Edamame and Quinoa Salad

Preparation Time: 10 minutes
Cooking Time: 15 minutes
Servings: 1 person
Ingredients:
- 1/2 cup cooked quinoa
- 1/2 cup shelled edamame
- 1/4 cup diced cucumber
- 1 tablespoon rice vinegar
- 1 teaspoon sesame oil

Procedure:
1. **Cook Quinoa:**
    - Cook quinoa according to package instructions.
2. **Combine Ingredients:**
    - In a bowl, mix cooked quinoa, edamame, and cucumber.
3. **Add Dressing:**
    - Drizzle with rice vinegar and sesame oil. Toss to combine.
4. **Serve:**
    - Serve immediately.

Macronutrients (approximate values per serving):
- **Calories:** 250 kcal
- **Carbohydrates:** 30g
- **Fat:** 8g
- **Protein:** 10g

Greek Yogurt and Berry Parfait

Preparation Time: 5 minutes
Cooking Time: None
Servings: 1 person
Ingredients:
- 1 cup Greek yogurt
- 1/2 cup mixed berries
- 1 tablespoon honey
- 1 tablespoon chia seeds
- 1 tablespoon granola

Procedure:
1. **Layer Ingredients:**
   - In a glass, layer Greek yogurt and mixed berries.
2. **Add Honey:**
   - Drizzle with honey.
3. **Sprinkle Seeds and Granola:**
   - Top with chia seeds and granola.
4. **Serve:**
   - Serve immediately.

Macronutrients (approximate values per serving):
- **Calories:** 250 kcal
- **Carbohydrates:** 30g
- **Fat:** 8g
- **Protein:** 20g

Lentil and Vegetable Stir-Fry

Preparation Time: 10 minutes
Cooking Time: 20 minutes
Servings: 1 person
Ingredients:
- 1/2 cup cooked lentils
- 1 cup mixed vegetables (bell peppers, broccoli, carrots)
- 1 tablespoon soy sauce
- 1 teaspoon olive oil
- 1 clove garlic, minced

Procedure:
1. **Sauté Garlic:**
   - In a pan, heat olive oil and sauté garlic until fragrant.
2. **Add Vegetables:**
   - Add mixed vegetables and stir-fry for 5-7 minutes.
3. **Add Lentils and Soy Sauce:**
   - Stir in cooked lentils and soy sauce. Cook for another 5 minutes.
4. **Serve:**
   - Serve hot over brown rice or quinoa.

Macronutrients (approximate values per serving):
- **Calories:** 300 kcal
- **Carbohydrates:** 40g
- **Fat:** 8g
- **Protein:** 15g

Protein-Packed Green Smoothie

Preparation Time: 5 minutes
Cooking Time: None
Servings: 1 person
Ingredients:
- 1 cup spinach
- 1/2 banana
- 1/2 cup almond milk
- 1 tablespoon almond butter
- 1 scoop plant-based protein powder

Procedure:
1. **Blend Ingredients:**
   - Combine all ingredients in a blender.
2. **Blend Until Smooth:**
   - Blend until smooth and creamy.
3. **Serve:**
   - Pour into a glass and serve immediately.
4. **Enjoy:**
   - Enjoy your protein-packed green smoothie.

Macronutrients (approximate values per serving):
- **Calories:** 300 kcal
- **Carbohydrates:** 30g
- **Fat:** 12g
- **Protein:** 20g

Quinoa and Black Bean Stuffed Bell Peppers

Preparation Time: 10 minutes
Cooking Time: 25 minutes
Servings: 1 person
Ingredients:
- 1 bell pepper, halved and seeded
- 1/2 cup cooked quinoa
- 1/2 cup black beans, rinsed and drained
- 1/4 cup corn kernels
- 1 tablespoon salsa

Procedure:
1. **Preheat Oven:**
   - Preheat oven to 375°F (190°C).
2. **Mix Filling:**
   - In a bowl, combine cooked quinoa, black beans, corn, and salsa.
3. **Stuff Peppers:**
   - Stuff bell pepper halves with the quinoa mixture.
4. **Bake:**
   - Place stuffed peppers in a baking dish and bake for 25 minutes. Serve hot.

Macronutrients (approximate values per serving):
- **Calories:** 350 kcal
- **Carbohydrates:** 60g
- **Fat:** 5g
- **Protein:** 15g

Tofu and Vegetable Stir-Fry

Preparation Time: 10 minutes
Cooking Time: 15 minutes
Servings: 1 person
Ingredients:
- 1/2 cup tofu, cubed
- 1 cup mixed vegetables (bell peppers, broccoli, carrots)
- 1 tablespoon soy sauce
- 1 teaspoon olive oil
- 1 clove garlic, minced

Procedure:
1. **Sauté Garlic:**
    - In a pan, heat olive oil and sauté garlic until fragrant.
2. **Add Tofu:**
    - Add tofu and cook until golden brown.
3. **Add Vegetables and Soy Sauce:**
    - Add mixed vegetables and soy sauce. Stir-fry for 5-7 minutes.
4. **Serve:**
    - Serve hot over brown rice or noodles.

Macronutrients (approximate values per serving):
- **Calories:** 250 kcal
- **Carbohydrates:** 20g
- **Fat:** 12g
- **Protein:** 15g

Vegan Chickpea Omelette

Preparation Time: 10 minutes
Cooking Time: 10 minutes
Servings: 1 person
Ingredients:
- 1/2 cup chickpea flour
- 1/4 cup water
- 1/2 cup diced vegetables (bell peppers, onions, spinach)
- 1 teaspoon olive oil
- 1/4 teaspoon turmeric

Procedure:
1. **Mix Batter:**
    - In a bowl, mix chickpea flour, water, and turmeric to form a batter.
2. **Cook Vegetables:**
    - In a pan, heat olive oil and sauté vegetables until tender.
3. **Cook Omelette:**
    - Pour batter into the pan and cook until edges are set. Flip and cook until golden brown.
4. **Serve:**
    - Serve hot with your favorite toppings.

Macronutrients (approximate values per serving):
- **Calories:** 300 kcal
- **Carbohydrates:** 40g
- **Fat:** 10g
- **Protein:** 15g

White Bean and Kale Soup

Preparation Time: 10 minutes
Cooking Time: 20 minutes
Servings: 1 person
Ingredients:
- 1/2 cup white beans, rinsed and drained
- 1 cup kale, chopped
- 1/2 cup vegetable broth
- 1/4 cup diced tomatoes
- 1 clove garlic, minced

Procedure:
1. **Sauté Garlic:**
    - In a pot, sauté garlic until fragrant.
2. **Add Ingredients:**
    - Add white beans, kale, vegetable broth, and diced tomatoes.
3. **Simmer:**
    - Bring to a boil, then simmer for 15 minutes.
4. **Serve:**
    - Serve hot with a slice of whole-grain bread.

Macronutrients (approximate values per serving):
- **Calories:** 200 kcal
- **Carbohydrates:** 30g
- **Fat:** 4g
- **Protein:** 10g

Chapter 5: Meal Plans

Welcome to Chapter 5, where we delve into the heart of the Metabolic Confusion Diet: customizable meal plans designed specifically for endomorph women. This chapter offers a variety of meal plans tailored to different caloric needs and dietary preferences, ensuring that you can maintain flexibility while adhering to the principles of metabolic confusion. By providing detailed meal plans for both high-calorie and low-calorie days, we aim to support your weight loss journey with practical, nutritious, and enjoyable options. Each plan is meticulously crafted to balance macronutrients and optimize metabolic function, setting the stage for sustainable success.

Meal Plan 1: Basic Alternating Schedule

Monday: High-Calorie Day (2000-2200 calories)

Breakfast:
- Avocado Toast with Poached Egg *(Pg.75)*

Morning Snack:
- Greek Yogurt Parfait with Granola and Honey *(Pg.92)*

Lunch:
- Chicken and Avocado Salad *(Pg.60)*

Afternoon Snack:
- Nutty Banana Pancakes *(Pg.77)*

Dinner:
- Baked Lemon Herb Chicken *(Pg.65)*

Tuesday: Low-Calorie Day (1200-1400 calories)

Breakfast:
- Berry Protein Smoothie *(Pg.55)*

Morning Snack:
- Cucumber and Hummus Bites *(Pg.71)*

Lunch:
- Grilled Salmon with Quinoa *(Pg.61)*

Afternoon Snack:
- Frozen Yogurt Blueberry Bites *(Pg.72)*

Dinner:
- Zucchini and Tomato Salad *(Pg.64)*

Wednesday: High-Calorie Day (2000-2200 calories)

Breakfast:
- Banana and Almond Butter Smoothie *(Pg.75)*

Morning Snack:
- Greek Yogurt with Honey and Walnuts *(Pg.72)*

Lunch:
- Lentil and Vegetable Soup *(Pg.62)*

Afternoon Snack:
- Protein-Packed Energy Balls *(Pg.73)*

Dinner:
- Quinoa Stuffed Bell Peppers *(Pg.67)*

Thursday: Low-Calorie Day (1200-1400 calories)

Breakfast:
- Avocado and Egg White Scramble *(Pg.55)*

Morning Snack:
- Dark Chocolate Dipped Strawberries *(Pg.71)*

Lunch:
- Shrimp and Zucchini Noodles *(Pg.62)*

Afternoon Snack:
- Kale Chips *(Pg.73)*

Dinner:
- Baked Lemon Herb Chicken *(Pg.65)*

Friday: High-Calorie Day (2000-2200 calories)

Breakfast:
- Scrambled Eggs with Smoked Salmon and Spinach *(Pg.79)*

Morning Snack:
- Berry Chia Pudding *(Pg.70)*

Lunch:
- Tofu and Broccoli Stir-Fry *(Pg.63)*

Afternoon Snack:
- Zucchini Muffins *(Pg.74)*

Dinner:
- Salmon and Avocado Salad *(Pg.68)*

Saturday: Low-Calorie Day (1200-1400 calories)

Breakfast:
- Chia Seed Pudding with Almond Milk *(Pg.56)*

Morning Snack:
- Spiced Roasted Chickpeas *(Pg.73)*

Lunch:
- Chickpea and Spinach Stew *(Pg.61)*

Afternoon Snack:
- Cucumber and Hummus Bites *(Pg.70)*

Dinner:

- Herb-Crusted Tilapia *(Pg. 67)*

Sunday: High-Calorie Day (2000-2200 calories)
Breakfast:
- Quinoa Breakfast Bowl with Spinach and Avocados *(Pg. 77)*

Morning Snack:
- Greek Yogurt and Berry Parfait *(Pg. 101)*

Lunch:
- Black Bean and Corn Salad *(Pg. 99)*

Afternoon Snack:
- Nutty Banana Pancakes *(Pg. 77)*

Dinner:
- Spaghetti Squash with Marinara Sauce *(Pg. 69)*

Meal Plan 2: 5:2 Schedule

Monday to Friday: Low-Calorie Days (1200-1400 calories each day)
Monday
Breakfast:
- Berry Protein Smoothie *(Pg. 75)*

Morning Snack:
- Cucumber and Hummus Bites *(Pg. 75)*

Lunch:
- Grilled Salmon with Quinoa *(Pg. 75)*

Afternoon Snack:
- Frozen Yogurt Blueberry Bites *(Pg. 75)*

Dinner:
- Zucchini and Tomato Salad *(Pg. 75)*

Tuesday
Breakfast:
- Avocado and Egg White Scramble *(Pg. 75)*

Morning Snack:
- Dark Chocolate Dipped Strawberries *(Pg. 75)*

Lunch:
- Shrimp and Zucchini Noodles *(Pg. 75)*

Afternoon Snack:
- Kale Chips *(Pg. 75)*

Dinner:
- Roasted Brussels Sprouts and Chicken *(Pg. 75)*

Wednesday
Breakfast:
- Chia Seed Pudding with Almond Milk *(Pg. 75)*

Morning Snack:
- Spiced Roasted Chickpeas *(Pg. 75)*

Lunch:
- Chickpea and Spinach Stew *(Pg. 75)*

Afternoon Snack:
- Cucumber and Hummus Bites *(Pg. 75)*

Dinner:
- Herb-Crusted Tilapia *(Pg. 75)*

Thursday
Breakfast:
- Cottage Cheese and Berry Bowl *(Pg. 75)*

Morning Snack:
- Apple Slices with Almond Butter *(Pg. 75)*

Lunch:
- Tofu and Broccoli Stir-Fry *(Pg. 75)*

Afternoon Snack:
- Greek Yogurt with Honey and Walnuts *(Pg. 75)*

Dinner:
- Spinach and Feta Stuffed Peppers *(Pg. 75)*

Friday
Breakfast:
- Kale and Spinach Smoothie *(Pg. 75)*

Morning Snack:
- Protein-Packed Energy Balls *(Pg. 75)*

Lunch:
- Lentil and Vegetable Soup *(Pg. 75)*

Afternoon Snack:
- Dark Chocolate Dipped Strawberries *(Pg. 75)*

Dinner:
- Quinoa Breakfast Bowl with Vegetables

Saturday: High-Calorie Day (2500-2700 calories)
Breakfast:
- Avocado Toast with Poached Egg *(Pg. 75)*

Morning Snack:
- Greek Yogurt Parfait with Granola and Honey *(Pg. 75)*

Lunch:
- Chicken and Avocado Salad *(Pg. 75)*

Afternoon Snack:
- Nutty Banana Pancakes *(Pg. 75)*

Dinner:
- Baked Lemon Herb Chicken *(Pg. 75)*

Sunday: High-Calorie Day (2500-2700 calories)
Breakfast:
- Scrambled Eggs with Smoked Salmon and Spinach *(Pg. 75)*

Morning Snack:
- Berry Chia Pudding *(Pg. 75)*

Lunch:
- Tofu and Broccoli Stir-Fry *(Pg. 75)*

Afternoon Snack:
- Zucchini Muffins *(Pg. 75)*

Dinner:
- Salmon and Avocado Salad *(Pg. 75)*

Meal Plan 3: Fitness Enthusiast Schedule

Monday (Leg Day): High-Calorie Day (2500-2700 calories)
Breakfast:
- Avocado Toast with Poached Egg

Morning Snack:
- Nutty Banana Pancakes

Lunch:
- Quinoa Breakfast Bowl with Spinach and Avocados

Afternoon Snack:
- Greek Yogurt Parfait with Granola and Honey

Dinner:
- Baked Lemon Herb Chicken

Tuesday (Rest Day): Low-Calorie Day (1200-1400 calories)
Breakfast:
- Berry Protein Smoothie

Morning Snack:
- Cucumber and Hummus Bites

Lunch:
- Grilled Salmon with Quinoa

Afternoon Snack:
- Frozen Yogurt Blueberry Bites

Dinner:
- Zucchini and Tomato Salad

Wednesday (Upper Body): Moderate-Calorie Day (1800-2000 calories)
Breakfast:
- Greek Yogurt Parfait with Granola and Honey

Morning Snack:
- Protein-Packed Energy Balls

Lunch:
- Tofu and Broccoli Stir-Fry

Afternoon Snack:
- Dark Chocolate Dipped Strawberries

Dinner:
- Herb-Crusted Tilapia

Thursday (Cardio): Low-Calorie Day (1200-1400 calories)
Breakfast:
- Cottage Cheese and Berry Bowl

Morning Snack:
- Apple Slices with Almond Butter

Lunch:
- Shrimp and Zucchini Noodles

Afternoon Snack:
- Kale Chips

Dinner:
- Spinach and Feta Stuffed Peppers

Friday (Full Body): High-Calorie Day (2500-2700 calories)
Breakfast:
- Scrambled Eggs with Smoked Salmon and Spinach

Morning Snack:
- Berry Chia Pudding

Lunch:
- Chicken and Avocado Salad

Afternoon Snack:
- Nutty Banana Pancakes

Dinner:
- Baked Lemon Herb Chicken

Saturday (Active Recovery): Moderate-Calorie Day (1800-2000 calories)
Breakfast:
- Quinoa Breakfast Bowl with Spinach and Avocados

Morning Snack:
- Greek Yogurt Parfait with Granola and Honey

Lunch:
- Tofu and Broccoli Stir-Fry

Afternoon Snack:
- Zucchini Muffins

Dinner:
- Salmon and Avocado Salad

Sunday (Rest Day): Low-Calorie Day (1200-1400 calories)
Breakfast:
- Chia Seed Pudding with Almond Milk

Morning Snack:
- Spiced Roasted Chickpeas

Lunch:
- Lentil and Vegetable Soup

Afternoon Snack:
- Cucumber and Hummus Bites

Dinner:
- Quinoa Stuffed Bell Peppers

Meal Plan 4: Professional and Busy Lifestyle Schedule

Monday: High-Calorie Day (2200-2400 calories)
Breakfast:
- Avocado Toast with Poached Egg

Morning Snack:
- Nutty Banana Pancakes

Lunch:
- Quinoa Breakfast Bowl with Spinach and Avocados

Afternoon Snack:
- Greek Yogurt Parfait with Granola and Honey

Dinner:
- Baked Lemon Herb Chicken

Tuesday: Low-Calorie Day (1200-1400 calories)
Breakfast:
- Berry Protein Smoothie

Morning Snack:
- Cucumber and Hummus Bites

Lunch:
- Grilled Salmon with Quinoa

Afternoon Snack:
- Frozen Yogurt Blueberry Bites

Dinner:
- Zucchini and Tomato Salad

Wednesday: Low-Calorie Day (1200-1400 calories)
Breakfast:
- Cottage Cheese and Berry Bowl

Morning Snack:
- Apple Slices with Almond Butter

Lunch:
- Shrimp and Zucchini Noodles

Afternoon Snack:
- Kale Chips

Dinner:
- Spinach and Feta Stuffed Peppers

Thursday: High-Calorie Day (2200-2400 calories)
Breakfast:
- Scrambled Eggs with Smoked Salmon and Spinach

Morning Snack:
- Berry Chia Pudding

Lunch:
- Chicken and Avocado Salad

Afternoon Snack:
- Nutty Banana Pancakes

Dinner:
- Baked Lemon Herb Chicken

Friday: Low-Calorie Day (1200-1400 calories)
Breakfast:
- Chia Seed Pudding with Almond Milk

Morning Snack:
- Spiced Roasted Chickpeas

Lunch:
- Lentil and Vegetable Soup

Afternoon Snack:
- Cucumber and Hummus Bites

Dinner:
- Quinoa Stuffed Bell Peppers

Saturday: High-Calorie Day (2200-2400 calories)
Breakfast:
- Quinoa Breakfast Bowl with Spinach and Avocados

Morning Snack:
- Greek Yogurt Parfait with Granola and Honey

Lunch:
- Tofu and Broccoli Stir-Fry

Afternoon Snack:
- Zucchini Muffins

Dinner:
- Salmon and Avocado Salad

Sunday: Low-Calorie Day (1200-1400 calories)
Breakfast:
- Cottage Cheese and Berry Bowl

Morning Snack:
- Apple Slices with Almond Butter

Lunch:
- Shrimp and Zucchini Noodles

Afternoon Snack:
- Kale Chips

Dinner:
- Spinach and Feta Stuffed Peppers

Chapter 6: Mindfulness and Stress Reduction Techniques

In the pursuit of weight loss and overall health, the role of the mind is as crucial as that of the body. Chapter 6 delves into the significance of mindfulness and stress reduction techniques in achieving and maintaining a healthy lifestyle, especially for endomorph women. Chronic stress and unmanaged anxiety can lead to hormonal imbalances, emotional eating, and disrupted sleep patterns, all of which can hinder weight loss efforts. This chapter explores various evidence-based strategies to cultivate mindfulness, reduce stress, and improve mental well-being. By integrating these practices into daily life, you can enhance your body's response to dietary and fitness regimens, ultimately supporting your journey towards a healthier, more balanced life.

Introduction to Mindfulness

Mindfulness, a concept rooted in ancient meditation practices, has gained substantial recognition in contemporary health and wellness paradigms. It involves the practice of bringing one's complete attention to the present moment, cultivating an awareness of thoughts, emotions, and physical sensations without judgment. This state of attentive presence can significantly impact one's mental and physical health, particularly in the context of weight management and overall well-being.

For endomorph women, who may face unique challenges in their weight loss journey, mindfulness can be a transformative tool. It helps in breaking the cycle of stress-induced eating, enhances emotional regulation, and promotes a more conscious approach to dietary and lifestyle choices. Mindfulness encourages individuals to listen to their body's signals, understand their emotional triggers, and respond to them in a healthier, more balanced way.

Scientific research supports the benefits of mindfulness, showing that it can reduce levels of cortisol, the stress hormone, which is often linked to weight gain, particularly around the abdomen. Moreover, mindfulness practices have been associated with improved sleep quality, reduced anxiety, and better overall mental health, all of which are crucial for maintaining a healthy weight and lifestyle.

In this subchapter, we will explore the foundational principles of mindfulness, its benefits, and practical ways to integrate mindfulness into daily routines. Whether through formal meditation practices or simple mindful moments throughout the day, adopting mindfulness can empower you to take control of your health, manage stress more effectively, and support your journey towards achieving and maintaining your desired body composition.

Benefits of Mindfulness for Weight Loss

Mindfulness, the practice of maintaining a moment-by-moment awareness of our thoughts, feelings, bodily sensations, and surrounding environment, offers a multitude of benefits for weight loss and overall health. For endomorph women, who often face distinct challenges in managing their weight, incorporating mindfulness into their daily routine can be particularly advantageous. Here, we explore the specific benefits of mindfulness for weight loss, supported by scientific evidence and practical insights.

Enhanced Awareness of Eating Habits

Mindfulness cultivates a heightened awareness of eating behaviors, allowing individuals to recognize patterns of emotional eating and unconscious snacking. By paying close attention to hunger and satiety cues, mindful eaters are more likely to make deliberate, healthier food choices and avoid overeating. This conscious approach to eating can significantly reduce calorie intake and support sustainable weight loss.

Improved Relationship with Food

Many individuals struggle with a complicated relationship with food, often characterized by guilt, stress, and emotional eating. Mindfulness encourages a non-judgmental attitude towards food, promoting a healthier, more positive relationship with eating. By fostering self-compassion and reducing food-related anxiety, mindfulness helps individuals enjoy their meals without overindulgence, leading to more balanced eating patterns.

Stress Reduction and Cortisol Management

Chronic stress is a well-known contributor to weight gain, particularly in the abdominal area, due to the release of cortisol, the stress hormone. Mindfulness has been shown to reduce stress levels effectively, thereby lowering cortisol production. By managing stress through mindfulness practices such as meditation, deep breathing, and mindful movement, individuals can prevent stress-related weight gain and improve their overall mental well-being.

Enhanced Digestion and Metabolism

Eating mindfully not only helps in controlling portions but also improves digestion and nutrient absorption. By chewing thoroughly and savoring each bite, the digestive system can function more efficiently, leading to better metabolism and energy utilization. This process supports weight loss by optimizing the body's ability to process and store nutrients.

Greater Enjoyment of Physical Activity

Mindfulness extends beyond eating habits and can also enhance physical activity. Mindful exercise involves paying attention to the body's movements, breathing, and sensations during workouts. This focus can make physical activity more enjoyable and effective, increasing motivation and adherence to regular exercise routines. For endomorph women, who may find it challenging to engage in consistent physical activity, mindful exercise can be a game-changer.

Long-Term Weight Maintenance

One of the most significant challenges in weight loss is maintaining the results over the long term. Mindfulness equips individuals with the tools to stay attuned to their body's needs, manage stress, and make healthier choices consistently. This sustainable approach to weight management reduces the likelihood of weight regain and supports long-term health and well-being.

In conclusion, mindfulness offers a comprehensive and sustainable approach to weight loss, addressing both the psychological and physiological aspects of eating and exercise. By integrating mindfulness into daily routines, endomorph women can achieve and maintain a healthy weight, improve their relationship with food, and enhance their overall quality of life.

Daily Mindfulness Practices

Incorporating mindfulness into your daily routine can be transformative, especially for those seeking to manage their weight and improve their overall health. Daily mindfulness practices help cultivate awareness, reduce stress, and foster a healthier relationship with food and exercise. Here are detailed practices that can be seamlessly integrated into everyday life.

Morning Mindfulness Routine

1. Mindful Breathing: Start your day with a few minutes of mindful breathing. Sit comfortably, close your eyes, and take deep breaths, focusing on the sensation of air entering and leaving your lungs. This practice helps center your mind and sets a calm tone for the day.

2. Body Scan Meditation: Before getting out of bed, perform a body scan meditation. Gradually bring your attention to different parts of your body, starting from your toes and moving up to your head. This practice increases bodily awareness and helps you identify any areas of tension or discomfort.

Mindful Eating

1. Mindful Breakfast: Dedicate time to eat your breakfast without distractions. Sit down at a table, savor each bite, and pay attention to the flavors, textures, and aromas of your food. Chew slowly and thoroughly, and notice your body's hunger and fullness signals.

2. Gratitude Practice: Before eating, take a moment to express gratitude for your meal. Reflect on the effort that went into preparing the food and the nourishment it provides. This practice fosters a positive relationship with food and enhances the eating experience.

Midday Mindfulness

1. Mindful Walking: Incorporate a short mindful walk into your lunch break. Focus on the sensations of walking—how your feet touch the ground, the movement of your muscles, and the rhythm of your breath. This practice helps clear your mind and reduces stress.

2. Mindful Listening: Engage in mindful listening during conversations with colleagues or friends. Give your full attention to the speaker without interrupting or planning your response. This practice enhances communication skills and fosters deeper connections.

Afternoon Check-In

1. Emotional Check-In: Take a few minutes in the afternoon to check in with your emotions. Sit quietly and observe your feelings without judgment. Acknowledge any stress, anxiety, or joy you may be experiencing. This practice helps you stay in tune with your emotional state and manage stress effectively.

2. Progressive Muscle Relaxation: Perform progressive muscle relaxation to release any physical tension. Sequentially tense and relax different muscle groups, starting from your feet and moving up to your head. This practice promotes relaxation and reduces stress.

Evening Mindfulness Routine

1. Mindful Exercise: Engage in mindful exercise, such as yoga, tai chi, or stretching. Focus on your breath, body movements, and the sensations you experience during the workout. This practice not only benefits physical health but also calms the mind.

2. Mindful Journaling: End your day with mindful journaling. Reflect on your experiences, thoughts, and emotions of the day. Write about what you are grateful for, any challenges you faced, and how you managed them. This practice encourages self-reflection and personal growth.

3. Sleep Preparation: Create a bedtime routine that promotes restful sleep. Turn off electronic devices, dim the lights, and engage in a relaxing activity such as reading or listening to calming music. Practice mindful breathing or a body scan meditation to unwind and prepare for sleep.

Integrating Mindfulness into Daily Activities

1. Mindful Chores: Transform routine tasks like washing dishes, cooking, or cleaning into mindfulness practices. Pay full attention to the task at hand, focusing on the sensations, sounds, and movements involved. This practice enhances mindfulness and makes mundane tasks more enjoyable.

2. Mindful Driving: While driving, focus on the experience of driving—notice the feel of the steering wheel, the sound of the engine, and the visual scenery. Avoid distractions and practice deep breathing at stoplights to stay calm and centered.

Incorporating these daily mindfulness practices can significantly enhance your overall well-being, reduce stress, and support your weight management goals. By consistently practicing mindfulness, you develop greater awareness and control over your thoughts, emotions, and behaviors, leading to a healthier, more balanced life.

Stress Management Strategies

Stress is an inevitable part of modern life, but its impact on health, particularly on weight management, is profound. Elevated stress levels can lead to hormonal imbalances, increased appetite, and a propensity to seek comfort in unhealthy foods. Therefore, effective stress management is crucial for achieving and maintaining a healthy weight. This chapter explores various stress management strategies that are not only effective but also easy to integrate into daily life. These techniques are designed to help you develop resilience, reduce stress-induced eating, and improve your overall well-being.

Understanding the physiological and psychological responses to stress is the first step in managing it effectively. Stress triggers the release of cortisol, a hormone that can increase appetite and lead to weight gain, especially in the abdominal area. Additionally, chronic stress can disrupt sleep patterns, decrease motivation for physical activity, and impair decision-making, making it harder to stick to a healthy diet and exercise routine.

The strategies discussed in this chapter are evidence-based and have been proven to help reduce stress levels. They range from physical activities, such as exercise and yoga, to mental practices like meditation and deep-breathing exercises. Social support and community engagement also play a vital role in stress management, providing emotional support and fostering a sense of belonging.

Each strategy is explained in detail, with practical tips on how to implement them in your daily routine. By adopting these stress management techniques, you can create a balanced lifestyle that supports your weight loss goals and enhances your overall health. Whether you are dealing with work-related stress, personal challenges, or the demands of daily life, these strategies will equip you with the tools needed to manage stress effectively and maintain a healthy, balanced life.

Breathing Exercises

Breathing exercises are a cornerstone of stress management and can significantly impact both mental and physical health. These exercises help regulate the autonomic nervous system, reducing the body's stress response and promoting a state of calm and relaxation. Here, we will delve into various types of breathing exercises, explaining their benefits and how to practice them effectively.

Diaphragmatic Breathing

Diaphragmatic breathing, also known as abdominal or belly breathing, involves engaging the diaphragm to achieve deeper breaths. This technique increases oxygen intake, promoting relaxation and reducing stress levels.

How to Practice:

1. **Find a Comfortable Position:** Sit or lie down in a comfortable position, ensuring your back is straight.
2. **Place Your Hands:** Place one hand on your chest and the other on your abdomen.
3. **Inhale Deeply:** Breathe in slowly through your nose, allowing your abdomen to rise while your chest remains relatively still.
4. **Exhale Slowly:** Exhale gently through your mouth, letting your abdomen fall.
5. **Repeat:** Continue this pattern for 5-10 minutes, focusing on the rise and fall of your abdomen.

Box Breathing

Box breathing, also known as square breathing, is a simple yet powerful technique used by individuals in high-stress professions, such as Navy SEALs, to maintain calm and focus.

How to Practice:

1. **Inhale:** Breathe in deeply through your nose for a count of four.
2. **Hold:** Hold your breath for a count of four.
3. **Exhale:** Exhale slowly through your mouth for a count of four.
4. **Hold:** Hold your breath again for a count of four.
5. **Repeat:** Continue this cycle for several minutes, adjusting the count to suit your comfort level.

4-7-8 Breathing

The 4-7-8 breathing technique, developed by Dr. Andrew Weil, is designed to promote relaxation and is particularly effective for falling asleep.

How to Practice:

1. **Inhale:** Breathe in quietly through your nose for a count of four.
2. **Hold:** Hold your breath for a count of seven.
3. **Exhale:** Exhale completely through your mouth for a count of eight, making a whooshing sound.
4. **Repeat:** Repeat this cycle four times initially, gradually increasing to eight cycles.

Alternate Nostril Breathing

Alternate nostril breathing, or Nadi Shodhana, is a yoga practice that balances the left and right hemispheres of the brain, enhancing mental clarity and reducing stress.

How to Practice:

1. **Find a Comfortable Position:** Sit comfortably with your spine straight.
2. **Close Your Right Nostril:** Use your right thumb to gently close your right nostril.
3. **Inhale Through Left Nostril:** Inhale slowly and deeply through your left nostril.
4. **Close Left Nostril:** Close your left nostril with your right ring finger, then open and exhale through your right nostril.
5. **Inhale Through Right Nostril:** Inhale through your right nostril, then close it with your right thumb.
6. **Exhale Through Left Nostril:** Open your left nostril and exhale through it.
7. **Repeat:** Continue this pattern for 5-10 minutes, focusing on your breath.

Benefits of Breathing Exercises

Physiological Benefits:

- **Reduced Heart Rate:** Slows down the heart rate, reducing the physical symptoms of stress.
- **Lower Blood Pressure:** Helps to lower blood pressure by promoting relaxation.

- **Improved Oxygenation:** Increases oxygen supply to the brain and body, enhancing overall function.

Psychological Benefits:

- **Enhanced Focus:** Improves concentration and mental clarity.
- **Emotional Regulation:** Helps in managing emotions, reducing anxiety, and promoting a sense of well-being.
- **Better Sleep:** Aids in falling asleep faster and improving sleep quality.

Incorporating breathing exercises into your daily routine can provide immediate stress relief and long-term benefits for your mental and physical health. These techniques are simple to practice, require no special equipment, and can be done anywhere, making them a versatile tool for managing stress effectively.

Guided Meditations

Guided meditations are structured meditation practices led by a guide or instructor, either in person or through audio or video recordings. These meditations provide direction and focus, making it easier for individuals to achieve a meditative state, especially those who are new to meditation. Guided meditations can vary in length and purpose, including stress reduction, relaxation, mindfulness, and even sleep improvement. Below, we will explore the benefits of guided meditations, types of guided meditations, and how to practice them effectively.

Benefits of Guided Meditations

Stress Reduction: Guided meditations help calm the mind and reduce the body's stress response by promoting relaxation and decreasing cortisol levels.

Enhanced Focus: These meditations improve concentration and attention by guiding the mind to focus on specific thoughts or imagery.

Emotional Balance: Regular practice helps regulate emotions, reducing anxiety and enhancing overall emotional well-being.

Better Sleep: Guided meditations designed for sleep can help relax the mind and body, making it easier to fall asleep and improve sleep quality.

Pain Management: Some guided meditations can help manage chronic pain by shifting focus away from discomfort and promoting relaxation.

Types of Guided Meditations

Mindfulness Meditation: Focuses on bringing awareness to the present moment, observing thoughts, feelings, and sensations without judgment. This type of meditation is effective for reducing stress and improving mental clarity.

Loving-Kindness Meditation: Also known as Metta meditation, this practice involves generating feelings of compassion and love towards oneself and others. It can improve emotional well-being and foster positive relationships.

Body Scan Meditation: Involves paying attention to different parts of the body, often starting from the toes and moving up to the head. This type of meditation is excellent for releasing physical tension and promoting relaxation.

Visualization Meditation: Uses guided imagery to evoke positive emotions and relaxation. Participants might visualize a peaceful scene, such as a beach or forest, to help calm the mind.

Breath Awareness Meditation: Focuses on the breath as a point of concentration. This type of meditation helps anchor the mind and improve focus.

Gratitude Meditation: Encourages reflection on things one is grateful for, promoting positive thinking and emotional well-being.

How to Practice Guided Meditations

Find a Quiet Space: Choose a quiet, comfortable place where you won't be disturbed. This helps create a conducive environment for meditation.

Choose Your Meditation: Select a guided meditation that aligns with your goals, whether it's stress reduction, improved sleep, or emotional balance.

Get Comfortable: Sit or lie down in a comfortable position. Use cushions or a chair for support if needed.

Focus on the Guide: Listen attentively to the guide's voice. Let the instructions lead your focus and attention, following the guidance without trying to control the experience.

Stay Present: If your mind wanders, gently bring your focus back to the guide's voice or the point of focus in the meditation. It's normal for thoughts to arise; the key is to return to the present moment without judgment.

Practice Regularly: Consistency is crucial. Try to practice guided meditations daily, even if it's just for a few minutes, to reap the long-term benefits.

Use Technology: There are many apps and online resources available that offer a wide range of guided meditations. Apps like Headspace, Calm, and Insight Timer provide accessible options for beginners and experienced meditators alike.

Practical Tips for Success

Set a Routine: Establish a regular meditation routine, whether it's in the morning, during lunch breaks, or before bed. Consistency helps build a habit and enhances the benefits.

Start Small: If you're new to meditation, start with shorter sessions, such as 5-10 minutes, and gradually increase the duration as you become more comfortable.

Be Patient: Meditation is a skill that develops over time. Be patient with yourself and understand that it's normal to have thoughts and distractions during practice.

Reflect on Your Experience: After each session, take a few moments to reflect on how you feel. Noticing the effects of meditation can reinforce the habit and motivate continued practice.

Incorporating guided meditations into your daily routine can offer profound benefits for mental and physical health. By providing structure and focus, guided meditations make it easier to achieve a state of relaxation and mindfulness, helping you manage stress and improve overall well-being.

Journaling and Reflection

Journaling and reflection are powerful tools for managing stress, enhancing self-awareness, and promoting emotional well-being. By putting thoughts and feelings into words, individuals can gain clarity, process complex emotions, and track their personal growth over time. This practice can be particularly beneficial for those undergoing lifestyle changes or facing health challenges, such as weight loss or managing chronic conditions.

Benefits of Journaling and Reflection

Stress Reduction: Writing about stressful events or feelings can help release emotional tension, reducing overall stress levels. This process allows for the externalization of worries and anxieties, making them feel more manageable.

Emotional Processing: Journaling provides a safe space to explore and understand emotions. By articulating feelings, individuals can better identify patterns in their emotional responses and develop healthier coping mechanisms.

Self-Discovery: Regular reflection helps individuals gain insights into their behaviors, thoughts, and motivations. This self-awareness is crucial for personal growth and can lead to more informed decision-making.

Goal Setting and Tracking: Journaling is an effective way to set and monitor personal goals. By documenting progress and setbacks, individuals can stay motivated and make necessary adjustments to their strategies.

Improved Mental Health: Research has shown that journaling can improve mental health by reducing symptoms of depression and anxiety. It serves as an outlet for expressing difficult emotions and provides a sense of relief and control.

How to Start Journaling and Reflection

Choose Your Medium: Decide whether you prefer a physical journal or a digital format. Some people enjoy the tactile experience of writing by hand, while others appreciate the convenience and accessibility of digital journaling apps.

Set Aside Time: Dedicate a specific time each day for journaling. This could be in the morning to set intentions for the day or in the evening to reflect on the day's events. Consistency is key to developing a sustainable journaling habit.

Create a Comfortable Space: Find a quiet, comfortable place where you can write without distractions. This will help you focus and fully engage in the reflective process.

Start with Prompts: If you're unsure what to write about, start with prompts such as:

- What am I grateful for today?
- What challenges did I face, and how did I handle them?
- How did I feel throughout the day, and what triggered those feelings?
- What progress have I made towards my goals?

Be Honest and Open: Write freely and honestly about your thoughts and feelings. Don't worry about grammar, spelling, or how your writing might be perceived. The goal is to express yourself authentically.

Reflect on Entries: Periodically review your past entries to reflect on your journey. Look for patterns in your thoughts and behaviors, and consider how you've grown or what changes you might want to make.

Techniques for Effective Journaling

Stream of Consciousness: Write continuously for a set period without worrying about structure or coherence. This technique helps uncover subconscious thoughts and feelings.

Gratitude Journaling: Focus on writing about things you're grateful for. This practice can shift your mindset towards positivity and improve overall well-being.

Mood Tracking: Keep a daily log of your mood and any factors that influenced it. Over time, this can help you identify triggers and develop strategies for managing your emotions.

Goal-Oriented Journaling: Set specific goals and use your journal to track your progress. Reflect on what's working, what's not, and how you can overcome obstacles.

Reflective Questions: End each entry with a question to ponder. For example, "What can I learn from today's experiences?" or "How can I approach tomorrow with a positive mindset?"

Integrating Reflection into Your Daily Routine

Morning Pages: Begin your day with three pages of free writing. This can help clear your mind and set a positive tone for the day.

Evening Reflection: Spend a few minutes before bed reflecting on your day. Consider what went well, what didn't, and what you're looking forward to tomorrow.

Weekly Review: Set aside time each week to review your journal entries. Reflect on your progress, challenges, and any recurring themes. This practice can help you stay aligned with your goals and make adjustments as needed.

Monthly Check-In: Conduct a more in-depth review at the end of each month. Evaluate your overall progress, celebrate your achievements, and set new goals for the coming month.

Journaling and reflection are invaluable practices for anyone seeking to improve their mental and emotional health, manage stress, and achieve personal growth. By regularly engaging in these activities, you can gain deeper insights into your thoughts and behaviors, develop healthier coping mechanisms, and create a more balanced and fulfilling life.

Conclusion

The journey towards achieving a healthier and more balanced lifestyle, particularly for endomorph women, is both challenging and rewarding. The principles outlined in this book aim to provide a comprehensive guide to help you navigate through the intricacies of the Metabolic Confusion Diet, tailored specifically for the unique needs and metabolic characteristics of endomorphs.

Summarizing the Core Concepts

Throughout this book, we have delved into the foundational aspects of understanding body types, particularly focusing on the endomorph. We've explored how the Metabolic Confusion Diet works, emphasizing the benefits of calorie cycling and the strategic management of macronutrients. These methods aim to keep your metabolism engaged and prevent the plateaus commonly associated with traditional dieting approaches.

Personalized Nutrition and Sustainable Habits

Personalized nutrition plays a crucial role in this diet plan. By crafting meal plans that cater to your specific metabolic needs and food preferences, you can ensure that your diet is not only effective but also enjoyable and sustainable. The emphasis on mindfulness and stress management, along with understanding and balancing hormones, adds another layer of depth to your wellness journey. These elements help in managing emotional eating and reducing the impact of stress on weight gain.

The Importance of Fitness and Community Support

Incorporating regular fitness routines, combining both cardiovascular and strength training exercises, is essential in transforming your body composition and improving overall health. The book also highlights the importance of building a supportive community. Engaging with others who share similar goals can provide motivation, accountability, and emotional support, which are critical for long-term success.

Monitoring Progress and Making Adjustments

Tracking your progress and being willing to adjust your strategies as needed is vital for continuous improvement. By regularly monitoring your achievements and challenges, you can refine your approach, ensuring that you stay on track towards your goals.

Final Thoughts

Transitioning from an endomorph to a more balanced body type requires dedication, patience, and a well-rounded approach. This book has aimed to equip you with the knowledge and tools necessary to make informed decisions about your diet, exercise, and lifestyle choices. Remember that each individual's journey is unique, and what works for one person may need to be adjusted for another. Embrace the process, celebrate your milestones, and stay committed to your health and well-being.

By adopting the Metabolic Confusion Diet and incorporating the seven pillars outlined in this guide, you are setting yourself up for a transformative journey towards a healthier, more balanced life. Keep this book as a constant reference and companion on your path to achieving your weight loss and health goals. With perseverance and the right strategies, you can overcome the challenges and enjoy the benefits of a fitter, happier you.

HERE IS YOU FREE GIFT!

SCAN HERE TO DOWNLOAD IT

Made in United States
North Haven, CT
13 September 2024

57362445R00070